# The Girls Who Refused to Quit

## *Volume 2*

To Tara ˣ

Keep leading by example
& shining your light! The
world needs more "Taras"...
with love & blessings
    Jen ˣ

        xxx

# The
# Girls Who
# Refused
# to Quit

*Volume 2*

*A Welford Publishing Collaboration*

Published in 2020 by Welford Publishing
Copyright © Cassandra Farren 2020

ISBN: Paperback 978-1-9162671-4-5

Front cover photograph © Guille Álvarez
Front cover design © Jen Parker
Author photograph © Kate Sharp Photography 2020
Editor Christine McPherson

A catalogue for this book is available from the British Library.

## Disclaimer

*This book is designed to provide helpful information on the subjects discussed. It is general reference information which should not be used to diagnose any medical problem and is not intended as a substitute for consulting with a medical or professional practitioner.*

*Some names and identifying details have been changed to protect the privacy of the individuals.*

*Poem written by Cassandra*

Your questions have no answers,
You feel lost, alone, and afraid.
Your head is spinning endlessly
As life passes in a daze.

It's time to trust your instincts,
Allow your pain and the darkness to fade.
Your lessons are ready to unfold now,
They will guide you day by day.

No anger or regrets will consume you
As you find the strength to move on.
Your voice and the strength within you
Were with you all along.

Hold your head high, live life on your terms,
You can do this, it's time to commit.
Know that you're worthy, take one step at a time

From
   *The Girls Who Refused to Quit*

# Contents

# Thank You for My Blessings

*Jennifer Bolton*

I stood alone in the kitchen looking down at the carving knife I'd just pulled from the wooden block. As I clenched it tightly in my hand, there was only one thought going through my mind… *One deep cut and it will all be over.* I could hardly see, as my eyes were drowning in the pain that was pouring from them. I could taste the tears as they were streaming down my face; my heart felt like it was going to jump out of my chest. 'I don't want this anymore!' I screamed.

After almost piercing my skin, I raised the knife up ready to stab myself through the middle of my wrist, fast and hard, so it would go straight through to the other side. No going back! The tears were still falling. I felt so utterly useless and not worthy of being on this planet any more, taking up space! I felt lost, hurt, sad, and confused. I was exhausted, absolutely broken, and drained emotionally, physically, mentally, and spiritually. I really didn't want to be here any more; I just wanted it all to end for good!

'Just do it, Jen, JUST BLOODY WELL DO IT!'

I started to feel numb. A darkness fell over me, wrapping itself around and engulfing me. You know when people talk about an angel on one shoulder and a devil on the other? Well, it was just like that, and the devil wanted to claim my soul.

Suddenly I was jolted back to reality… I heard myself screaming, 'What the hell am I doing? What the fuck! Don't be so fucking stupid!' My mind was racing. What about Danny? I've got a son; how could I leave my boy? *What the hell's wrong with me?* But I just wanted something to take away the unbearable pain. It had all got too much, and I guess I didn't really know what else to do.

I visualised him walking in and finding me there on the floor in a pool of blood, wrists slit, and my dog Milly sitting by my side. Oh, how could I be so selfish? I quickly dropped the knife and my knees buckled beneath me. I fell to the floor and held my head in my hands, sobbing. Over and over I kept thinking how on earth my life had come to this.

Everyone thinks I'm so strong, usually the joker and so confident. A strong, funny independent woman. Well, I used to be, but not any more. And certainly not now.

Milly, my beautiful little dog daughter, came over and licked the tears on my cheeks, and I hugged her tightly and thanked her for being there. I was scared and in shock at what had just happened. *How could I be so bloody selfish?* I thought. *What stopped me, though?*

As I sat on the kitchen floor still sobbing, I heard the song *Don't Worry About a Thing* playing on the radio. I hadn't heard anything other than my own thoughts up until that point. This had to be a sign. Bob Marley's *Three Little Birds* is one of my favourite songs and has been for many years, but since 2015 it's had a much deeper meaning to it. I knew this was my mom telling me everything was going to be alright, that dropping the knife was the right thing to do, and this wasn't my time.

The hairs on the back of my neck stood up as I gave thanks to my beautiful mom, as well as thanking God, Source, The Universe, Buddha, a Higher Presence, whatever's your preference. I was extremely grateful to still be here and receiving this message. It was a blessing. And it had such impact because my beautiful mom was no longer here; she was dead! Loulou, as we affectionately called her, had gained her wings on Easter Bank Holiday Monday, 2015. She was now my angel in Heaven.

Oh, how I longed for a Mommy hug right now. I might be in my fifties, but I just wanted my mom to hold me and make me feel safe, like she used to. Maybe that's why the song *Three Little Birds* is so poignant for me; it's like a lovely warm hug off my mom whenever I hear it. The power of physical touch is incredible, and hugs are so important. I'm happy to say our family has always been very tactile, from being kids through to adults. Hugs, and kisses, and I love you's… we had lots of them. All blessings.

It was only four years before that my mom had died, but we lost her long before her physical death. I will never forget the day she looked me straight in the eye and said, 'Ooh, who are you?'

I felt my heart drop to the pit of my stomach and my legs turned to jelly. I wanted to cry, but I smiled and said, 'It's me, Jenny, your daughter.' After that, I never said it again. I realised I'd lost her.

'Oh, I know who you are, you're that nice lady from down the road,' Mom replied.

I had always known it would happen someday, but that knowledge doesn't make it any easier when it actually happens. That day, my heart broke into a million pieces, right there. After researching about vascular dementia, I quickly realised that we have to enter their world as they can no longer survive in ours. I tried to keep Mom in my world, but I had to enter hers.

I first noticed things were changing with Mom when the taps were left running or she'd burn the pans when cooking, then the front door would be left open. It didn't all happen at once, but things did build up quite quickly. She was losing her sight, too, which frustrated her. She had always loved reading and doing crosswords, but this soon stopped.

To watch my beautiful mom become swallowed up and disappear into this cruel disease, vascular dementia, was traumatic and devastating. It seemed to come out of nowhere, yet the signs had been there for a while. Hindsight's a great thing, isn't it? We only lived two minutes away and Mom would regularly pop round for a cuppa, but more and more frequently she'd forget which was our door. Danny found her wondering outside the wrong house one time, and she was so confused, bless her. Things were clearly getting worse.

I soon realised that it was no good saying, 'You know who I am' or, 'I told you that earlier' to someone with dementia; they can't comprehend this any more. They are not trying to be awkward or annoying; this is their reality. Keep things simple is what I learnt, and 'love lies' became a big part of keeping Mom reassured.

She would say, 'I want to go home. I want my Mom.'

Some people might reply, 'Well, you can't, you haven't got a mom any more. She died years ago.' But that would just upset and stress her, so I found it best to say, 'We'll see her later, ok?'

Sometimes we'd have a long discussion, other times not, but I learnt to sense her mood and go along with it.

Mom would say, 'Oh, we're going to see her later then?'

Me: 'Yes.'

Mom: 'Oh, ok, that's good.'

Me: 'So, shall we go and have a cup of tea and a singsong?'

Now she might say the same thing 100 times some days, but she was always happy and reassured with the answer. She was in a happy loop. As I said, these love lies were all from the heart and told with love.

Someone said once that it was wicked not telling Mom the truth. But she/they (people with dementia) don't understand, and it's not their fault. Their brain cells are dying! I/we do understand, so it's our responsibility to keep them feeling reassured and safe. I would often tell her she was safe, and that helped, too. I could only imagine what she was thinking sometimes when I saw the sheer terror in her eyes. It was all very real to her, much like being a child. In fact, people suffering from this horrible disease are like toddlers, and that's how I looked at Mom. Our roles had reversed; I was now the parent and she was the child.

Fortunately, I managed to capture many magical moments on camera and video, and I am so grateful to have them all to look back on. We all are. They are wonderful, cherished moments, beautiful blessings.

During her illness, we were all living with anticipatory

grief – also known as living grief. We were grieving the parts of Mom that were already gone, as well as a loss of dreams and what might have been. At the same time, we had to handle changing family roles; all sorts, really. We were grieving both our parents, knowing they were already on their journey home.

I wanted to learn all I could about what was stealing my mom away bit by bit. Lots of information can be sourced on the internet from dementia experts, like the amazing Teepa Snow. I did some printouts for myself and the family, and gave them this information with a kind heart, trying to help keep us all consistent in our caring, so that we would not confuse our beautiful mom. I was keen to share the information that I'd found was helping me. Sharing is caring, after all.

Mom loved singing, and that's probably where I got it from. In fact, all us girls would sing with our folks when we were younger. Music played a big part in all our lives, and these are some of my happiest memories.

We'd sing along to Doris Day, and Andre Rieu and his orchestra. There were others, but towards the end it was mostly these two she wanted to hear. We rejoiced in our singing and used to love harmonising together, but when Mom reached a stage where she couldn't do the harmonies any more, I realised things were changing.

Eventually, as things got worse and Mom struggled with the stairs, we had a hospital bed put in the front room, with a single next to it so we could stay overnight to look after her. We were already on a rota doing daily shifts but would sleep over now, as well as caring for Loulou and Pops.

In 2014, I managed to organise having the garage turned into a wet room to make life much easier for everyone, as Mom was registered blind and the stairs were now a no-go. The risk of falls was high, and both parents were regularly in and out of hospital with various problems. They were never left alone, though. One of us would stay at the hospital, another at home, and I am incredibly proud of how we all cared for our parents. I really am.

There will never be the right words to describe what it was like caring for our folks. Dad was very poorly with end stage heart and kidney failure; he was on dialysis 3-4 times a week for 4 hours at a time, which really took its toll. Our whole lives had changed. We would take it in turns to take him and pick him up. Eventually, it got too much for Mom when we went there, and she became bored and agitated, so one of us would look after Mom and another stay with Dad until he was comfortable to stay alone.

The dreaded day came when Mom gained her wings and left her physical body. She looked like a beautiful little doll laying there. I'd painted her nails the day before with her favourite pink. My heart completely shattered as I watched my beautiful mom take her last breath. I was dying inside, but trying to hold it together for my dad whose heart was breaking right in front of me. He was holding Mom on the bed and sobbing.

Witnessing my dad, my hero, crying for the woman he had spent sixty years with, broke me even more. I felt like I shouldn't be watching this private moment between husband and wife as life was ending, but I'd asked Dad if he wanted me to leave and he'd said he wanted me to stay with him. I was grateful to be there for both of them.

Mom's passing was actually quite beautiful, if there's such a thing. There was soft music playing and a sense of calm in the air. It was very peaceful.

But I couldn't believe she had really gone, that I'd never be in her presence ever again. I'd never hold her hand, hug her, brush her hair (very delicately), sing and dance together, or make her giggle when I'd say, 'Chuck it in the fuck-it bucket' about stuff! She'd always laugh, 'Ooh, you are a naughty girl!'

My mom was the most amazing and incredible woman. I'm sure many people feel this way, but I feel so honoured to have been her daughter, and will treasure the memories we shared over the years – both before and after I became a mom myself. We used to love singing 'Oh Danny Boy…' to Danny when he was still growing in my womb, and of course once he was born.

Obviously spending so much time at my folks' house impacted on my and Danny's relationship, but I thought he was doing much better than he actually was.

I remember my dad saying thank you to Danny, some time after Mom had gone, for sharing me with him. Looking back, I honestly don't know how we did it, but we did. I was just getting on with everything as best I could, but really struggling with my own health issues. Not realising, though, that my son was struggling, too.


## January 2017

I had a radical hysterectomy with some complications, and after surgery I stayed at Dad's house to recover.

Milly was so good, and Dad would call her 'the bab', his little dog granddaughter, bless him. She is a natural healer and has brought great comfort to all of us throughout the years, and especially Dad. He adored her.

## *September 2017*

Nine days after his 83rd birthday, Dad left us. It wasn't as peaceful as Mom's passing, but I was with him at the end, along with my sisters. And he was where he wanted to be – at home, in his chair. It all happened quite quickly really, and he wouldn't let go of my hand.

Watching your parents die changes you; it's something you can't un-see. Being with both my folks as they took their last breaths, I feel, are blessings. I had sung softly to Mom as she was leaving us, and held her hand as she lay with Dad holding her on the bed. Now it was Dad's time; he was sat upright and looking straight at me. His defibrillator was going off, which was traumatic, but I smiled and said, 'You're alright, Dad, everything's ok… Go to Mommy.'

My sisters were all talking, too, but for a time I couldn't hear them. It was just me and my hero, as I watched the light fading in his piercing blue eyes. I almost lost it completely when I saw a solitary tear rolling down his cheek, but somehow I managed to hold my own tears back until he'd taken his final breath. My whole body was trembling inside as my heart broke once again into a million pieces. Pops had gone. I was now an orphan; that was honestly how I felt.

13 days later, Jennylou, my 34-year old niece and

goddaughter, gained her wings. We were burying Dad just 4 days later.

A massive tsunami of shock, disbelief, and grief continued.

Having faced many challenges over the years, including depression, anxiety, bullying, mental and physical abuse, disability, and being raped on my seventeenth birthday, I've learnt that it's through these tough times that we truly grow mentally, physically, and spiritually.

I'm still working on myself holistically, embracing meditation, mindfulness, Reiki, and other amazing tools for wellbeing. Music, though, is my therapy. I have songs and stories to share, and healing to do. I live the attitude of gratitude every day and want to be of service, helping as many people as I can.

I know I am stronger for turning my pain into purpose, and will hopefully inspire Danny and others to find their purpose through adversity, and just maybe we can all help make the world a better place. By healing ourselves, we become healers of others, and by doing so we heal the planet. How amazing is that!

I admit I feel vulnerable sharing all this, so why am I doing it?

To quote Cassandra Farren, 'Do not allow the ghosts from your past to steal the happiness of your future.'

I'm freeing myself from all of the ghosts of the past, right back to my childhood. I am reclaiming my power!

There are lessons in absolutely everything, including our blessings, and I feel blessed to be here on earth at this unique time. More and more people are living consciously and embracing mindfulness, which is wonderful.

So, look out for lessons in your blessings. And that inner power we all have? Let it grow and guide you. We are all capable of great things once we put our hearts and minds to it. Grief and almost ending my life proved this to me.

I finally reached the point where I was ready to talk to Danny about that day when I'd come so close to ending it all. Our relationship had broken down drastically in the last couple of years, and neither of us was coping. I was eating and drinking my emotions, and we were both smoking way too much after burying Dad and Jennylou close together.

That's when he opened up and said he'd failed at suicide, too. OMG, I was absolutely mortified. I thought I was going to throw up!

I felt such a failure as a mom. Had I paved the way for my son, by living with and trying to navigate through my depression all of his life. I thought I'd done better than that. Angst, shame, and guilt were churning inside of me. But somehow, I pulled myself together and, with tears of both pain and relief streaming down my face, we hugged each other tightly for the first time in a long time.

I obviously hadn't realised how much everything had impacted Danny. Not just the deaths of his beloved Nan, Grandad, and cousin, but throughout his young life, bless him. With mental health now being recognised more openly at last, it's so very important to be honest with ourselves and each other.

I was so thankful that my darling boy had failed at suicide, too. It was as though we were both being given a second chance, as well as an insight into each other's heart and soul, the angst and turmoil. We truly empathised with each other, and at last there was light outshining the dark.

Later that night, as we carried on talking, I felt a real deep connection on a soul level. We hadn't been this close in a very long time and it was beautiful, exactly what we both needed. As we discussed all sorts, Danny admitted that he'd like to be an inspirational speaker and I can see this manifesting with his wonderful words of wisdom. He is an old soul with much love to give.

I looked at him and said, 'Son, we are obviously still here for a reason. Maybe you're going to help your generation and I'm going to help mine. Let's lead with love, and shine our lights together.'

## *Poem written 26/12/15*

For Mommy x
Been thinking about you…
I've missed you today.
So, I got an old photo
And kissed it to say,
'Although you're not here,
In body you've gone,
Your love, warmth, and spirit
Will always live on.'
I miss how we'd dance
And we'd sing every day.
We'd always be giggling
The bad days away.
'You're that lovely lady,
I know you, my friend.'

'I'm actually your daughter.'
But I learnt to pretend
And entered your world
Of invisible things,
Memories, and siblings,
Your favourite things.
The nightmares, the turmoil
Such horrible fears.
'You're safe, I won't leave you.'
'Oh, thank you, my dear.
You make me feel safe.
Jen, I love you so much.'
'I love you more, Lucy.'
And so miss your touch.
What I wouldn't give
For one last Mommy hug
Although…

# A message to my younger self...

If I could go back in time and speak to my younger self, I would give her a big hug and say you are loved, and you are perfect exactly as you are.

It's not your fault the things that happened to you, so stop blaming yourself for being taken advantage of.

You are enough; always were, always will be. You will learn and grow through each experience, as you question yourself and your worth, but try not to over-analyse and be so hard on yourself. Know that you have the strength and courage to overcome anything.

You are authentic, beautiful inside and out, with a big, kind heart that sees the good in everything. Keep this safe, it's a precious gift. Learn to really love yourself as you do others, for you are worthy and a child of the Universe. You belong here, so make the most of absolutely everything. Be proud of all you've overcome, and embrace what's on its way. Keep smiling and believing in yourself, and never apologise for being you; you are authentic and, yes, emotional, but you will learn to navigate through it all for you are a natural healer and empath. Try not to become cynical and keep faith in mankind; there are good people out there. Keep shining your light, being kind to others, and being true to yourself. Strive to be happy.

I wish I had known sooner that our thoughts and words are so much more powerful than we realise. Our words become flesh, and thoughts become things.

Being able to survive everything I have been through has shown me that its ok not to be ok. There is purpose and meaning in the world which is generated through love. I am ever thankful for my life, for love, and for my many blessings. I am exactly where I'm meant to be at this present moment in time. I now feel that there is so much more to life. I have found my soul purpose and I want to help and inspire others to find joy in every day. To turn pain into purpose and loss into light, leading with love.

How others see us doesn't define us or who we are. We are so much more. We can all be beacons of light and hope for others to find their way in the dark.

I am love, I am presence, I am here now.

I am open and receptive to all the good and abundance in the Universe.

I am thankful, I am blessed, I am strong, I am safe. I am brave, I am courageous, I am powerful, I am a warrior, I am the divine feminine, I am woman, I am a goddess, I am a queen, I am grateful, I am stoic, I am unique, I am amazing, I am beautiful.

I am me, and I am free.

*I am The Girl Who Refused to Quit.*

## Dedication

Danny,

I know the last few years have been testing to say the least. I just want you to know how proud I am of how you've got through it all.

I truly believe, though, this last year we have grown immensely, both individually and together with all we've gone through. I am so proud to be your mom and so very sorry for not being there when you needed me most. I have learned so much from you, I really have. So, thank you for that, my darling.

I see you, I hear you, I appreciate you with all my heart for your love and support. I hope you know I am here to love and support you, too. We are a team. We always have been, it's just life and circumstances got in the way and blurred our vision for a while.

You are a beautiful and special soul, Danny. You have such depth and wisdom, an inner strength and glow, a bright light that has dimmed at times through no fault of your own, but is so bright I hope the rest of the world gets the chance to see it. Shine your light all over and live your best life, my beautiful boy.

I love you to the moon and back, son. Always have, always will, no matter how old you are or how tall you grow. You are my most precious blessing of all. Xxx

## About the author

Jennifer was born and lives in Birmingham, England with her son Danny & dog daughter Milly. She is a lightworker, passionate about helping others & strongly committed to self-development, healing & spiritual growth.

Jen has been described as a heart centred fun loving soul with the voice of an angel and heart of a lion. An earth mother and soul sister to many. Jen is an accomplished singer/songwriter and TV actress.

When not singing she can be found spreading blessings of love & positivity. Jen feels honoured to be part of this book & is currently writing her life story "Thank You For My Blessings".

Jen truly cherishes time spent with family and friends.

Her mission is to share her story and her voice with the world, empowering people to love themselves enough to never give up on life. Helping them to turn their pain into purpose & loss into light.

Live, love, laugh & be happy!

# Contact

jenniferboltonofficial@gmail.com

www.jenniferbolton.co.uk

For FREE MP3 players & bespoke music for people living with dementia please contact norrms@gmail.com

(Founder of The Purple Angel Dementia Awareness Campaign)

Please support "The Angels Will Listen" Purple Angel Charity song written by J Bolton N McNamara J Purser available on iTunes Thank you

All proceeds go to The Purple Angel Dementia Awareness Campaign.

# The Courage to Be

## Kerlin Sabogal

I will never forget the day someone told me my voice did not matter. I was eleven years old, living on a tiny island in the Colombian Caribbean, with few resources, and a small, unfinished house.

I grew up in a loving family, where our first language was Spanish. Education was everything to me, and my only hope to have a better future was to work hard at school. I would try to get A's at school by giving my best, but for some reason my English teacher could not see my potential. Every time I attended the class, I felt defeated, ashamed, and questioned whether I would ever be good enough to fulfil all my big dreams and goals. I felt like a failure, but nobody knew it; I never said it. Why wasn't I good enough to learn a new language like others? Why would my own teacher allow others to bully me? Those were always the questions that followed me around like a ghost for many years.

My parents always taught me to work hard, laugh often, and to keep my word. They encouraged me to use my voice, but often I would ask myself how I could use my voice if every time I went to school, I felt like I did not have one.

Instead of crushing my dreams, though, my teacher's cruel words became my inspiration to always fight harder and to work tirelessly. That's when I decided that I would achieve a degree in a language other than mine, and not just any degree – a Master's degree. I promised myself that nothing was going to stop me, not her words, not my circumstances, and certainly not my background. That proved to be the defining moment which would shape the course of my life. Courage and determination were key to where I wanted to go, so off I went!

Over the years there were many times I felt things were not going my way, and that my path was continually blocked by outside forces. Despite the challenges, I knew that how I responded to the things that happened to me would be the difference between a life of despair or a life of hope.

You would think that a little girl in my circumstances would not have so much hope for the future. But for as far back as I can remember, I always had a positive force and determination bigger than myself. It was this strong internal knowing that gave me hope, and it continues to do so. Courage and hope have always been the guiding lights in my life – ones that have never gone out, even in my darkest days. I had so many doubts and questions, but against all the odds I graduated with Honours from high school and accepted a 5-year scholarship at a private university in Colombia!

Yes, it was a great accomplishment... but not the one I wanted.

I was still haunted by those voices that put me down and told me learning a new language was going to be almost impossible. I achieved my degree in journalism, but I promised myself that, no matter what, I would leave my country as soon as I graduated. I knew I had a bigger dream to fulfil.

In January 2008, I started my journey to get a visa to the United States, which proved to be no easy task.

The visa for a low-income family in Colombia is almost impossible to get, and once again life showed me there was a bigger force that wanted me to understand I was good enough.

In the end, though, I got the visa – after my parents emptied their savings accounts, and I sold all of my books, my computer, and pretty much everything else I owned, in order to pay for my immigration process. Yes, I sold everything. After all, I had a big dream to fulfil, right? And like Eckhart Tolle said, 'Life is an adventure, not a package tour.'

I was determined to embark on this unknown adventure, but how would I survive in a new country without knowing anyone? Good question! I told myself I would figure it all out when I got there. I wasn't afraid, because I believed I was one step away from bringing one of my biggest dreams to life. I was sure that as soon as I got to that new country, I would immediately learn English and show everybody back home what I was made of.

## *Autumn of 2008*

The first African American was going to be president of the most powerful nation in the world, the United States of America. Barack Obama won the 2008 Presidential race and showed the world that 'it doesn't matter where we come from', but it does matter where we choose to go. I mention this because I arrived in America when things were changing, and so was my life. It wasn't a coincidence. I believe life is always speaking to us, so I knew life was trying to tell me something. I felt hope was with me.

I saw a sign through my window on the airplane, *Welcome to JFK international airport!* I was in the capital of the world! I couldn't believe it. My mom always used to tell me that I was rarely impressed by something, and she was right! But when I stepped into New York city, I was definitely in a *Wow!* mood. I was impressed by literally everything.

My adventure in New York did not last too long. I took a 2-month course that allowed me to learn some basic English and I met wonderful people there – some of whom are lifelong friends now; almost family. And although I struggled learning the language, people were always kind. Instead of laughing at my accent or bullying me, they taught and helped me. In fact, I became friends with a Japanese guy, and since our language was a barrier (he did not speak English, either), we used his translator to communicate while attending our basic English classes. I was learning, but not as quickly as I wanted. Some days were full of excitement, but others were full of anxiety and tears.

In the middle of this process, I met a new partner, and for a short time I became a victim of an abusive relationship. At that time, I thought that was better than being alone in a big city. But I was wrong! It's better to stand alone than to have someone that tears you apart. I was trying my hardest to achieve my dreams, but life kept throwing challenges at me.

Thankfully, I found people that supported me, and with their help, I left that relationship. I continually questioned myself: Had leaving my homeland been worth it? Was going back maybe an option? Could I make it in a place where I did not know anyone or, even worse, nobody knew who I was.

Usually, in times of uncertainty my mind would advise me not to do anything and eventually I will find an answer. But this time, I did not have time to wait for that answer… I was in the United States of America, I had no choice but to make it happen, and going back home was NEVER an option. I had a lot of things to prove to myself and one of them was that I could live my life fearlessly.

Two months of class were almost at an end and I wanted to continue learning. A family friend from Colombia told my mom that I could go to Houston, Texas, as it was a great state and would offer me new opportunities. So, I listened to my mother, grabbed the only suitcase I had, and made the decision to move. Once again I was setting off on an adventure, going to another big city where I had no clue what was in store.

Fear is a powerful and conveying emotion, and yes, I was afraid to start in a new city. But as I read once, 'You become what you believe, not what you wish for or what you want. You become what you expect in your heart.' And I knew my heart was always leading me to achieve my goal.

It was a sunny day when I arrived in Houston. A relative from that friend welcomed me, and I had a place to stay for two weeks – four weeks maximum. After that, I would be on my own. I started working to save some money, and little by little I started building my life. I had very broken English, but I tried my best to practise every time I could.

There were other things that worried me, though. I needed to learn to drive and to find a permanent place to live as soon as I could. Two months passed, things started to take shape, and I got not one but two jobs! Every day I worked from 7am, sometimes through until midnight, taking the bus to get to work.

In the mornings, I worked helping Cuban refugees, and in the afternoons, I sold women's underwear at one of the Victoria Secret stores. I worked hard and kept learning English with the help of my co-workers. Every scenario of my life at that moment was a learning experience, and I grabbed them with both hands.

After a few months of feeling a little more stable, I enrolled in English classes and planned to take one semester before trying to sit my TOEFL (Test of English as a Foreign Language) exam. Passing this exam would allow me to enrol into the Master's program so, as you can imagine, I was so excited about this English class.

I started doing my assignments and, as always, I tried hard. I spent hours reading the vocabulary and writing sentences in order to learn. But to my surprise, I came across the same type of teacher I'd had when I was eleven years old. Here I was in another country, at the age of 24, and being bullied by my teacher again. When I asked her one day if she thought after the completion of the course I would be ready to take the international test that would allow me to go into graduate school, she said I wasn't ready. And that it would take a long time for me to get my Master's.

The TOEFL test requires a certain score in order to be accepted into Graduate School in America. I remembered the same feeling I'd had when I was eleven years old and asked myself if this perhaps was a sign. Why was I still experiencing the same situation I'd had thirteen years earlier?

From that moment on, I started studying harder, determined that her words would not break me. In fact, they made me, and against all odds I took the test three months later. To her surprise, I passed the test and I had the score I needed to enrol in the Master's program.

Two months later, after a long interview and English test, I was accepted into the Master's degree in Bilingual Education. It proved to me that I needed to listen to that voice inside me, that force that never left me.

At that point, I thought my life was almost perfect. I had met a wonderful guy, who I married and had a son with. My English was still broken, and he did not speak any Spanish, but somehow we made it work. We bought the house of our dreams, and I was about to start my Master's degree! Life was good for once, and I was finally living the American dream. Little did I know my dream was about to collapse in a big way.

Suddenly, I found myself in the middle of a stressful divorce, while pursuing my degree. I'd thought I had made it, but my dream had turned into a nightmare. I prayed on my knees every day, desperate to find an answer. I did not understand why my life could collapse in such a way.

My first year of the Master's was almost over when my academic counsellor sat me down and suggested that, due to the stress, I should stop the program. She was concerned that the divorce process could affect my academic performance and eventually ruin my semester. I refused to let this situation stop me, though. Nothing was going to come between me and my goals.

We all have storms to face, but what looks like a setback can often be a beautiful turning point. It was hard to see it at the time, but a couple of years later I realised that my divorce saved my life and made me the woman I am today. The pain blindfolded me for a while so that I couldn't see the rainbow in the clouds.

As you might expect, I did not accept the suggestion from my academic counsellor, and I enrolled in four more classes the next semester, determined to finish before my son's 5th birthday. I had made myself a promise to graduate before that date and I was so close that nothing was going to stop me, not even a painful and complicated divorce.

The new journey in front of me wasn't easy. I was a full time Master's student, I had a 4-year-old with me, and I worked part-time, so my income wasn't enough. But I had been taught to honor my word, so I started preparing to get my life back on track.

As the day of the graduation was fast approaching, I remember crying while writing my final dissertation paper for my last class. My life was crumbling in front of me, but on the other hand I knew I had a purpose. I was honoring a promise I had made to my son and to my younger self.

## *May 13th, 2017*

A day I will never forget. It was a beautiful day; the sun was shining, and the clouds were clear. It was my Master's graduation day, and my induction into the International Honor Society of Education. I was graduating with honors – something I had not expected.

That day was a mixture of emotions. I did it; I had the diploma with me! That young 11-year-old girl that I had once been was there in spirit. I'd honored my word throughout all these years. But the most important part of all was that I was graduating on time, before my son Terry's 5th birthday. I graduated May 13th – his 5th birthday was the following day. So, right on time.

After that magical day, my life began to change. I started a new full-time job working in education – one of my passions – and I took up three new hobbies – traveling, yoga, and running. Little by little, I started picking up the pieces to complete my own new life-puzzle. I started traveling solo around the world in my free time, which opened a new perspective on life and gave me a life purpose.

As far back as I can remember, I always knew I wanted to make a difference when I came to America. With this thought in mind, I pursued a career in Bilingual Education and completely dedicated my efforts and time to work in projects to help young people at risk. As English is not my first language, I wanted to help immigrant students who, like me, felt isolated or misplaced because they had an accent or didn't know the language. I became the mentor I did not have when I was in middle school, knowing that would make a difference to so many young people.

Wanting to make a difference beyond classrooms, I took trips to discover the world and also to work in some of the most impoverished countries on the planet. It was such a huge turning point in my life. I was not only fulfilling my purpose, but I had started shaping a new dream.

## November 2019

I became the founder of an educational organization called The Courage to Bee. This name means a lot to me, because it took courage for me to learn a new language at the age of 24, after years of being bullied as a teen by my own language teacher. Taking the risk of traveling solo, becoming a single mother, and starting a new career from scratch, also took some courage.

They say courage is not the absence of fear; courage is being afraid and doing it anyway... And I did. So, this project is dedicated to helping kids to find hope, courage, and trust. In the end, that is everything I needed when I was their age.

Through all these years, I have planted the seeds to live a life with hope. The energy of hope can help us veil fear in uncertain times; it helps us build trust to move forward. I have found my greatest hope in the space of gratitude and I believe the more grateful you are, the more hopeful you become. I have realized that gratitude was expanding my courage and my sense of happiness. Appreciating what we have in life changes our personal vibration. We must celebrate every step and every act of courage we take.

Today, I celebrate every act of courage I have taken.

On the road to achieving my dreams, many things were lost but many other amazing ones were gained. Although I know the world might be a little harsh from time to time, I try to accept everybody with compassion because they are living a journey I might not know about.

I celebrate every day of my life, knowing I am making a difference, like many wonderful people around me. As one of my favourite writers said, 'I am only one, but I am one. I can't do everything, but I can do something. And because I can't do everything, I will not refuse to do something that I can do.' So, with courage, I am doing my part, honoring that 11-year-old me. Because it DOESN'T matter where we come from; it DOES matter where we choose to go.

# A message to my younger self...

If I could go back in time to speak to my younger self, I would tell her with compassion and love not to be so hard on herself, but to move with the current of life and not try to control it. I would tell her not to be scared to lose, or she would end up losing herself in the process. I believe courage flourishes when you are in the flow of life and makes you feel free. All you need is to move with the flow of life, literally. Fighting or resisting the current won't take you anywhere.

I would tell her to enjoy every moment as if it was her last. If we have the idea that this is the only moment we have, we could enjoy more of what's happening in the now, rather than having a point of arrival. One of my favorite writers, Deepak Chopra says, 'The point of arrival is NOW.' It took me years to understand this. I thought I would be happy when I achieved this or have that, which made me lose focus in those precious moments I was living. I was waiting, always living for the future. And when we get there, sometimes we don't recognize it because we are not completely present to enjoy it. We miss some moments because we don't truly show up.

If I could go back in time, I would tell her that constantly showing up for herself and others will take her to where she is now, and that resilience, hope, and courage would be the three words that she should carry with her always. We don't realize that we don't live life; life lives us. And we must live in our truth, whatever that means to each one of us. Most importantly, we must live in gratitude and know that LIFE is the dancer and we are the dance.

It takes commitment to oneself and others to experience results in our lives, but that's a choice we made every day when we woke up.

Are you showing up for yourself and others? Are you enjoying the NOW of life, while working on your dreams? Without missing what the present moment is bringing you?

Ask yourself these questions and start being a DOER. Our dreams are valid and we must have them, but remember that dreams without action are solely thoughts or words. Putting action into them is a decision we make every day. We MUST.

I am a courageous woman who will fight to fulfil her dreams; the one who knows there is always a light at the end of the tunnel.

*I am The Girl Who Refused to Quit.*

## Dedication

To my son Terry to always find courage to pursue his dreams, not matter what! To my parents, brother and two best friends (Marleny & Evelyn) for believing in me and their unconditional love and support.

## About the author

Kerlin holds a BA in Journalism and corporate communication and Master's in Bilingual Education. She has called Texas home for the last 10 years, but has taken much pride in being an island girl since she was born and raised on an island in the Colombian Caribbean!

When she came to the United States at 24 years old she completely dedicated her efforts and time to work in bilingual education & projects that help youth at risk!

English is not her first language so she wanted to help immigrant students like her that have felt isolated or misplaced because they have an accent or don't know English.

Kerlin is the founder of The Courage to Bee, a project close to her heart. With this project she is touching and building the life of many students in Latin America (first pilot project is on the works in the beautiful Country of Dominican Republic).

Since turning 30 she has dedicated her free time to practice meditation & running! She learned that the best way to get good at something is DOING it! So she did!

In the end, she values and firmly stands by living

in GRATITUDE as that is the key to living a life of contentment and happiness!

## Contact

www.thecouragetobee.com
Facebook and IG page @thecouragetobee
Email Ksabogalhou@gmail.com
Thecouragetobeeproject@gmail.com

# To Rise Again

## *Sea Rakaisau*

*How did I get here?* My skin is numb and clammy from the wave of exhaustion engulfing me like fire in this very moment. Hot flushes, dizziness – confused – desperate – surreal. *But why?* As I look out across the room, all I can see are familiar faces. This is a very real experience (*yes, Sea, it is really happening*) yet I cannot reconcile how I am feeling.

I am sitting here as the woman of the moment at a reception. A wedding reception. I am the BRIDE at her own wedding reception, full of the promise and potential youth has to offer –yet I am adorned with humiliation, feeling more weak and overcome than I have ever been in my 22 years of life. I look down from my place at the top table on stage, to see half of the guests seated against the backdrop of a half empty room. The stage, on which I sat, would become my only sense of elevation that day.

*How did I get here?* would become the lyrics to my life's soundtrack – recurrent, recalcitrant, and rebellious – with each echo of my failures successively lodged in the fibre of my skin that would sing me to sleep for the next five years.

So, how did I get here?

Let me set the stage.

For as long as I can remember, I have lived a transient life. By the time I finished high school, I'd attended sixteen schools in 5 different countries, some of which I attended twice. For the most part, it was adventurous, and in hindsight it was a way to fast-track resilience within a child. Except that eliciting resilience, as opposed to teaching resilience, produces fragmented life skills – you start something but never finish it. You make a new friend and become close, then suddenly, you're on the move again. Soon, a friend is only a friend in that moment. For that chapter. Making and breaking friendships becomes a normalised cycle. That's if I had the chance to say goodbye, but most, if not all of the time, I was unaware of my own departure. Or I didn't have enough time to make real friends who would have cared when I left.

Children who grow up experiencing some kind and level of trauma tend to show the world what is happening to them in the most inconvenient and infamous ways. Some children or young people lie about their realities, others create superficial connections because they anticipate moving on again, and some enter the juvenile justice system. The effects of adverse experiences can be so powerful that they can form the basis of long-term, unhealthy relationships, habits, and behaviours. And this is what you have to work with to find acceptance in the world. You will take any sign or form of acceptance – even though you have no idea what that looks like.

This type of backdrop is a perfect set-up for imagination to set in like wildfire, and before long, two parallel realities are concurrently in motion. Well, one is reality and the other is your preferred 'reality'; your fantasy – something that is especially unlikely to happen. Fantasising that you are in a safe, warm home with a fridge full of food. Fantasising that your partner loves you. Fantasising that I wasn't in this situation and that I would wake up from this nightmare!

There is a term for this type of fantasised life in psychology, and that is dissociation. It can show up in different forms, depending on the person and their circumstances, but essentially it's when someone 'checks out' of their reality because the present moment they're dealing with (or not) has become a trigger in itself. A dissociated state of being is when you are physically present but mentally travelling and traversing through an alternative 'reality' in your mind, because your only form of acceptance and safety is found there – in your mind.

Dreams are often grand and filled with hoped-for things. Dreams are a bonus to your actual and lived reality. It often becomes a seed for your future goals and visions and, more importantly, it is here in our dreams that we begin our journey towards our purpose, with each step closer being well thought-through and well resourced.

But what if your dream was to be in your dream, instead of in your reality? That is when my eyes opened – when it was too late!

When my eyes opened, I was looking down to a half empty wedding reception room, filled with only half of the love and half of the support I thought I had. That one moment justified my whole life spent with dissociation as my crutch, because my only dream and purpose was to survive. My soul was buried under the rubble of shame and pain I had collected over the years, that seared my senses, and I could not push against the remorse. It was as if I'd stepped into my episode of *This is Your Life,* but could not recognise the corridors I had built in my own reality.

Here I was, in what is meant to be the day of every girl's dream – marrying Prince Charming – yet this is the moment where fantasy and reality amalgamated. Each sequential thought revealed the tragedy and the deceit of these exchanges. I suddenly integrated with reality and I was only 'seeing' my life.

Growing up was adventurous but also arduous. There were a lot of challenges and heartbreaks, but there were also a lot of memorable and joyous occasions. And for this very reason, reflecting past behaviours and exploring its roots can prove difficult.

It can lead to a sense of guilt to tell your story, because if you do, it can upset people you love, care about, and admire. But this is *your* story. Your experiences are valid and unique to you, and though carers may create experiences for you, they cannot control how you experience them. Growing up, there was a common practice for children to 'be seen but not heard', which is mainly to do with learning cultural protocols by observing. However, the implicit approach creates a sense of invisibility – to be hidden, and preferably unheard. It is important to explore these themes appropriately and with relevant support, particularly if it is inhibiting parts of your story and yourself to be heard, as it perpetuates guilt.

This guilt is something I had to let go of in order to reconcile my past, and to move forward in my present and future with the acceptance that I am not overriding and negating wonderful memories. It means I can share my story without fear of feeling triggered to the point of dissociation. Rather, it means I have taken the lessons learnt and can apply them, like self-compassion, in real time. I no longer have to hide in a virtual, concurrent world to validate me and why I am here.

What if you choose someone who is actually a good person? Someone who possessed some fundamental core values that you could aspire to, respect, and appreciate? As I looked down to the half empty room, rinsed of love and support, I was seated next to someone who had been a great friend for years and someone I had respected, but all I could think about was running away.

And I did. In my mind.

I spent the entire reception dissociated from the reality of what was happening before me. And why, you may ask, do I keep referring to the half empty room, rinsed of love and support? It's because at that very time, two realities were concurrently being played out. Half of the reception was live and active in the reception venue with the entire wedding party. The other half held their own reception party at a different venue.

I hadn't seen my father for quite a while. Our relationship existed through tolerance during that time. But that day, I desperately wanted to reach out to him to tell him that this was something I did not want to do. For once, I wanted and needed my father to rescue me.

I remember walking down the aisle, tears streaming down my face, grieving in my spirit, desolately dismal, and my trusted long-time companion – dissociation – could not help me. I tried to check out, but my body was mournful, howling to the heavens – to anyone, someone out there,

'Hear me, please!' I was in a church full of people, but none of them could help or save me from myself. My spirit was so distressed that the ceremony was paused. My Pastor halted the proceedings to pray for peace upon me, giving me a chance to regulate myself. Imagine, if I had taken that as a window of grace? Imagine if I had known what grace was, at that point in my life! I was so lost, I wished I could be teleported to Mars.

Seated at the reception head table, I was not as emotionally distressed. We'd just returned from taking photographs, and that meant spending time with my best friend – my sister. My siblings are my regulators, and they would go on to live with me until their own independence. Their presence proved a comfort to me during my – what would be from this reception moment – five-year valley.

But here is the thing about unresolved trauma. It has wicked, awkward, and unpredictable timing to show up and take over. What do you do when your eyes open inside a tsunami?

By this time, the pores on my skin only had receptors for safety. Whatever safety looked like, whatever protection felt like, I would be attracted to that. It didn't have to make sense; it just had to feel safe and protected or similar, just to get me through a bout of shame that was trying to take over me.

Growing up in my day, a common currency was honour and shame. This was generally the hard and fast rule. You either performed to honour, or brought shame to yourself and, ultimately, the family. It wasn't something that had to be spoken about or explained, because it was part of the ecology. Each day I would be led by the shame in my skin;

each night, soft pillows would fold me into regret; and in the morning, this cycle would reset.

When survival is a person's baseline, their tolerance window is vulnerable to any perceived threats, and keeping myself safe was my baseline. Every day would melt into the next, and as survival lined the purpose of each day, it eventually accumulated to 5 years.

Consistency and predictability are the two main pillars that create safety. A safe mindset, safety in a relationship, safety to build trust, and some level of safety to take risks. Children and young people who become adults with adverse experiences have an ability to recreate chaotic relationships and circumstances, because that is familiar to them. It is the lesser of two evils, because it is a 'known' and therefore a 'safe' bet. It is familiar territory to navigate, which reduces protective behaviours, given their sense of danger and tolerance towards what can be considered at-risk situations but to them are normal.

I looked to my husband seated next to me at the head table, completely unaware of the emotional turmoil I had been experiencing the whole time. He continued to celebrate with his good friends and his loving family, whilst I remained deluged and disconnected, occasionally giggling with my sister seated on my other side. I forced myself to do the rounds, taking pictures at the tables with guests and obliging customary rituals, but by the end of the reception I was so emotionally exhausted, there was nothing left to drain. I just wanted to sleep for the rest of my life. Like my childhood experiences of being preferably unheard, today I dreamed for this day and me to be forgotten.

No-one would argue that he was and is a good person

who loves his children unequivocally. Our first date had been seven years before that day. And throughout the seven years of relationship, he was reliable, loyal, and caring, and he extended these qualities towards my siblings. Why wouldn't I be with someone who's been there for me in ways that mattered?

Having lived a transient life, a lot of gaps were revealed in my behaviours, and that created another set of problems. These gaps showed up in my educational life, my basketball life, and my life in general. But despite being a person full of gaps and adverse experiences, I found someone who represented safety. His family accepted me from the moment we met, and I was intrigued to feel invited and interesting enough to get to know. This also meant that my innocence made me naïve when making informed decisions.

An interactive home setting was not familiar to me, but acceptance to me, at the time, was sharing meals, talking and laughing with one another, watching movies together on a Saturday night in, and telling each other 'I love you'. Suddenly I was experiencing a different template and I was paying attention. Through the lens of trauma, a warm light can feed hidden desperation, hurling false hope into full force, setting off a game of blindfold chess – only this time it's your life.

How does it not make sense to build a life with someone I'd grown up with and whose family accepted me unconditionally? Who was I to question and be ungrateful for where I was? It could be worse, right? I wrestled with this question because of the true ethical paradox I was facing. How does someone find their voice, let alone find value in their voice, when its girded by shame, humiliation, and unforgiveness? It became apparent to me that every life choice leading up to sitting at that reception table had been made out of deficit.

Unresolved trauma, compounded by trauma-induced life decisions, is a recipe for disaster. And it all came to a head for me five years down the track, because unfortunately there is a saying, 'You can run but you can't hide.' Seeds that had been planted and watered over time had reached crisis point, and as my eyes opened, I was surrounded by a monster jungle no thanks to dissociation negating real life circumstances.

By the fifth year of marriage, our relationship had reached a critical point, and we found ourselves at a crossroads. I had suggested reconciling our situation through counselling, but in the end I attended alone. When you're experiencing a valley and the only tools you have to survive are shame, fear, and regret, your spirit starts to search for answers in the most unusual, mysterious, and extraordinary ways.

*What if I used my fear to fuel my fire?* Granted, a small fire, but it began to warm me up. This was the turning point. My soul made demands on my potential and prompted a self-belief that I could take shame, fear, and regret, and use them to my benefit. I would face this head-on, embracing it and allowing myself to understand the authority I had surrendered to. Now it was time to take that back.

Curious and ready to explore, I found a trickle of power that would propel me to prosperity. I began to entertain (not dissociate) what life would be like without the burden of shame: *I mean, what if?*

Once hope anchored itself inside my spirit, it did not let go! I felt like I had finally buckled into the right vehicle for my journey. I anticipated rough terrain ahead, but I sensed this was the way out of the conditions I had been living under. It would not be easy, but I knew I had to set off on this season of my journey, and trust that it would all work out whether my relationship was intact or not.

Given loyalty and acceptance were important qualities to me, I prayed a prayer of faith. I made a spiritual bond, allowing myself a two-year period to reconcile all differences. Despite the obstacles – the length and severity of them – I would honour my bond and do everything I could to remedy the situation, to forgive, and to move forward. For two years, despite some heavy and heart-wrenching, at-risk situations, I finally reconciled my promise and honoured every detail and process before going my separate way.

And it was in this moment that I found out that falling out of love can be just as euphoric as falling in love.

Whilst my strength unearthed, I did not feel like a new woman or person. I focused on being worthy to know myself all over again. I was now in the position to own and rewrite my story; to establish my true identity that was not dictated by trauma or penned by the hands of other authors.

In the first year of singledom, I was promoted three times with three pay rises; moved into a bigger home and car, and enjoyed the freedom to enjoy it all with my family, for the first time in my life without shame, fear, or regret. For once, in that moment in time, I was able to celebrate who I am without adorning myself with the opinions of others.

I did not share my separation with my own family until two years later. My promise during the last two years of my relationship was to reconcile as much as possible, which I honoured, but then I decided to extend that process towards my former in-laws. During this time, I focused on the family I had known for fourteen years. Separation involved everyone, and it was important to keep the family relationships intact. I would spend the next two years building and remaining in close contact with his family, because they were a strong part of my life, and will continue to be so for my children.

After two years, I told my family that I was single and, suffice to say, it was received with a bit of shock but also disappointment at the possibility that I had not felt I could talk about it. However, I was able to share that during such a life-altering transition, it was important that I had kept the voices in my head (my support network) clear and meaningful, and not allow myself to be distracted from the task and purpose ahead of me.

Fast forward to now, a lot has changed with my relationship dynamics – some for the better, and some for the better in other ways. A significant moment was when my ex-husband and I called a meeting with the children to apologise to them for failing to keep our family together, for not fighting harder, and for not being emotionally available to them during that time.

We now have an open-door policy whereby if they want to ask any questions, to resolve any unspoken beliefs and thoughts, we will be there for them to unload. Lessons and healing furnish resilience, and with that comes hope. No matter how far down the road you may find yourself, with a blueprint version of your life you can still choose change in the face of adversity.

Have faith in your ability, and allow yourself some grace to grow, moment by moment.

# A message to my younger self...

If I could go back in time and speak to my younger self, I would want to tell her to choose self-compassion over judgement.

To trust in your faith. But more than that, remember you have always been accepted by your creator. I would desperately explain that although resources and support seem limited to you, they are not as far away as you think. Keep searching, keep digging deep – what you are looking for is within reach, and each time you reach out, you succeed!

I wish I had known I was truly enough. That I did not have to try to find myself and what I needed in others, in circumstances, and in things. I wish I had known that communication and transparency would have saved me from so much disappointment and despair.

Being able to survive everything I have been through has shown me that anything is possible. It has taught me not to ignore my gut feeling but to explore it, and to explore the resources available to me, from my faith to my friends. Even my foes can teach me a thing or two.

There is no limit the soul cannot find that the light cannot touch.

I now feel as if I am still learning and evolving, but I

continue to make demands on my potential because I have experienced what that can produce!

I am Sea Rakaisau.

*I am The Girl Who Refused to Quit.*

## Dedication

To Latai, Arieta and Sam, thank you for walking with me, throughout all my seasons.

## About the Author

Sea, who lives in Sydney, Australia, has been described as a 'wise, discerning hurricane!'

Sea is passionate about development work with marginalised communities and people affected by conflict and natural disasters. When she's not immersed in development work or grant writing proposals, Sea can often be found chasing sunrises, sunsets and God sized dreams.

For Sea, contributing to this book, during a pandemic was a God sized dream.

A polymath and spoken word poet, Sea actively creates performance platforms for untold stories, to be heard. A firm believer of second chances, Sea's neuro-leadership skills harnesses evidence-based practices as a vehicle to usher in change, grace, forgiveness, self-compassion, wholehearted living, acceptance, resilience and mastery through the written word and spoken word.

Sea's mission is to inspire new thought-leaders who champion meaningful change on every level in all walks of life. No matter where you are in life, you can re-write your story, you can change your trajectory and you can flourish and thrive in new beginnings.

Sea's vision is to inspire you to rise again.

## Contact

E-mail: sea@writeme.com

# Letting Go
## *Judith Ward*

I stared down at my feet on the bare wooden floorboards and glanced around the barren living room. In that moment, I had never felt so sad and alone. *Was this it? Was my life destined to be one big failure after another?*

I had risen early that morning and watched the dawn creep in slowly, as if it sensed how unwelcome it was. I had been dreading this day for many months. As the sunlight crept into the room, it slowly came into focus, like a photograph developing.

The sun didn't inject much warmth into my body, but still I wished I could freeze this moment forever. I gazed out of the bay window onto the quiet London cul-de-sac that I had loved so much. I watched the autumn leaves falling from the trees, forming a carpet of rust and auburns.

I wasn't ready. I needed more time. I didn't want to start all over again. Why did everything have to change at once?

All the pictures that had once lined the walls in the lounge were now gone. The fireplace was bare. It was an empty shell once again. My whole life and everything I had cherished was now packed away in boxes – photographs of my friends who lived around the corner; keepsakes from my career. And now I had to say goodbye to my home that I loved dearly.

Soon the removal men would come, and then it would be time to close the door on this chapter of my life forever. Everything that I had come to know as security was crumbling before me.

This wasn't meant to happen to me. I'd had my whole life mapped out before me. I had moved to London from Northern Ireland twenty years before as a young, fresh-faced university graduate. London was vibrant and exciting to me, and I felt privileged to move there. Back then, I couldn't wait to discover what new, exciting adventures and opportunities were awaiting me. I imagined myself living in the hub of all the action in the city, embracing the buzz of London life, walking down the famous iconic streets, observing strangers on the underground, visiting bars and restaurants, and having a career I loved.

On paper, I had it all, and I had worked so hard to get there. I had studied for years and worked various jobs until I landed my dream job in television. I had dreamt about this all those years ago when I was that shy girl at school. My job was to support behind the scenes on high-profile Saturday night productions. I was recognised as being hard working, and after a few years I was given more responsibility and became an advisor to freelancers working on shows with traumatic story lines. I loved it. I was able to give talks to the production teams, and I supported the freelancers I worked with.

In my personal life, I had a fantastic circle of friends who lived around the corner and I lived in a home that

I loved. It was a simple terraced house, but it had all the old features like sash windows, high ceilings, and original fireplaces, and was set in a sleepy cul-de-sac surrounded by lovely neighbours. Most importantly, it felt like home to me. I had a beautiful six-month-old daughter, and this was her home, too.

And then I found myself uttering four words one evening…

'I want a divorce.'

These four words created a powerful explosion which would completely change the trajectory of my future.

That evening, time stood still. I glanced at the smiling images staring back at me from picture frames on the fireplace, and I knew in that moment my life was never going to be the same again. My heart began to race, my palms became sweaty, adrenaline rushed through me, and my mind was racing. It felt like I was going to have a panic attack. *Had I made the right decision?*

I raced upstairs to my bedroom and collapsed on my bed in tears. I loved my home and I didn't want to say goodbye to the life I had worked so hard to build. But my life as I knew it was over. I was distraught!

I wrapped myself around a pillow on my bed and the tears began to flow. There was a whimper and I wondered where it had come from, and then I realised it was me. I had never felt so alone as despair poured out of me in those moments. My body and heart ached, and I felt like I had fallen into a dark pit. My diaphragm felt constricted and painful, and when I exhaled out came a flood of tears. It was as if the grief and emotions that had been buried deep for months were at last being released.

The sobbing continued for a while, and eventually I closed my eyes and allowed myself to switch off from this nightmare. There were so many questions running through my mind. *What was going to happen? Where was I going to live? How was I going to navigate all of this on my own as the mother of a six-month-old child?*

When eventually I awoke, I looked outside the sash bedroom window that lined the front of the house and noticed the sun was setting. It was still warm, but the sun now hung lower in the sky. Some lights had been switched on in a neighbour's house, casting a warm glow across the street. I glanced at the magnolia tree in his garden and I remember how beautiful it was when it was in full bloom. It was absent of flowers right now, and in this present moment it felt representative of my life – barren of hope, and with no promise of blossoming again. Another neighbour was taking out his bin, and a little grey cat crossed the road slowly. Life was going on for the rest of the street. I had walked along that road so many times, pushing the pram with pride… and now everything was changing. I wondered if things would ever be the same again.

I made a phone call to my parents and the floodgates opened again. I choked my words out and felt like such a failure and that I was letting them down. We had only got married just over a year ago, and I remembered all the expectations and money that had been put into the wedding. My parents lived in Northern Ireland, so I could not drop round and see them easily. I longed to have a hug that evening.

When I checked in on my daughter that night, I heard her sleeping contentedly and knew then that I had to keep going for her. I hadn't expected or anticipated myself being in this position. As I reflected on my past life and experiences over the last ten years, I wondered if I was repeating the same pattern over and over again. Was I destined to make the wrong choices and have a life of struggle? I needed to keep going to carve out a future for both my daughter and me.

In the months that followed, I felt like I was caught in the eye of a storm. I felt battered and bruised, clinging to the wreckage of my life, and each new attack left me breathless. The fallout from those four words radiated for months to follow. My emotions swung like a pendulum. One moment I was sad and grieving for my old life, the next I was feeling lost and abandoned.

Everything I had built up was falling apart. I loved my London life, but I found it impossible to make it work on my own. I found myself in a dark place. Anxiety, fear, and uncertainty kicked in. I felt as though I was going round and round in circles. Going back to work was not an option. I didn't have a typical 9-5 job; my job now required travel, and local nurseries were very strict on pick-up times. I did my calculations and realised that with London childcare costs of £80 a day, a mortgage and living expenses, I would only be taking home £25 a month if I returned to work full time. My options had become limited!

Every day felt like a struggle. I was living on adrenaline, I couldn't sleep, and I felt alone and full of self-pity. I knew that I needed to find something flexible so that I could be there for my daughter while she was growing up. I explored some different career options with a lady from work, as I had indicated that I was going to have to leave. I looked into so many different options, but I knew I wanted to be able to help others as part of my future.

A friend mentioned that she knew someone who had retrained as a hypnotherapist, so I decided to try it for myself. I was curious and a bit scared of the unknown, but I went to see a lovely local lady hypnotherapist in London. I went for one transformational session and this had me hooked. I left feeling calmer and more relaxed. I had an idea… maybe I could make this work for me? I did some research and enrolled in a London training school which was highly recommended to me as the gold star for hypnotherapy. For the first time in ages, I felt excited about my future!

When I started doing the classes, I learned about the brain, and it felt as though a light bulb had been switched on. I now knew and understood my brain and why I was feeling the way I did. I had further hypnotherapy sessions during my time at the college and it helped me to learn so much about myself, to understand my strengths, and how to manage negative thoughts and anxiety. I was able to sleep, feel calmer, and get through the day-to-day nappy changes, tidying the home for house viewings, responding to solicitor paperwork, whilst trying to find somewhere to live.

I had to learn to cope with the knowledge that my security blanket was slipping. My life felt like a stack of dominoes, and once that tumbling momentum started, it just kept going and I didn't know how to stop it…

My beautiful home that I cherished and had spent years working towards was being sold from under me, and I would be homeless with nowhere to go. I tried so hard to make it work by staying, but in the end I had to surrender to the fact that it was not sustainable for me, both financially and emotionally. The only option available was to go back home to Northern Ireland to my parents' house, and into my old childhood bedroom.

I awoke from my daydream of the last eight months and took one last glance around my empty living room. Small beams of light crept through the wooden blinds and I watched them for a moment as the light caught little specks of dust. And then I came back to reality with a thunderous crash.

This was it. All my dreams, plans, and life goals were now side-lined. I had never felt such a failure. I thought I had moved on since I was that shy girl at school. Soon I would be leaving to go to the airport with my mum and young daughter.

I heard the sound of the van arriving outside and greeted the burly removal men at the front door. My belongings were loaded into the van, and they set off. My house felt hollow, and the empty rooms echoed. We packed our hand luggage and the child seat into the car then I closed the front door for one last time. I dropped my set of keys through the letterbox.

With a heavy heart, we made the journey to Heathrow Airport. Driving through familiar streets and past the local shops made me feel sad, but I kept a brave face and didn't cry. The only pinprick of light in the gathering darkness was the thought of seeing my family and returning home to living by the sea, as I had always loved its calming effect.

As the plane took off and circled London one last time, I said a mental goodbye to my old life. This time, I had a one-way ticket… It was final. I kept myself focused on my daughter during the flight and looked around at all the passengers, listening to the familiar accents. I was on my way home after being away for all of my adult life.

As the taxi drove up my parents' driveway, I caught my breath and realised I had been functioning on autopilot all day. There had been something surreal about the journey home.

Now I breathed in the fresh sea air. I felt the blustery breeze on my face as I walked up to the front door. I looked at the view of the beach in front of the house, and saw the waves crashing onto the shore. In the golden light of the dipping sun, a shadow in my heart spread across my body and gave me a chill. I told myself I would have to adjust; I'd need to turn my back on the chapter of my London life and start a new one. I had my course in London to finish, and would have to carve out a new life for me here.

My parents said I would always have a home for the two of us, which made me feel welcomed and safe. But that evening, in bed in my old bedroom, I glanced round at my flowery wallpaper, my old desk, and a few well loved, old teddy bears, and I sobbed tears for my past. I felt like such a failure.

The first few days went by slowly, as if time was dragging its feet. My thoughts kept turning to London and my old life. My feet felt heavy and reluctant, and I was still afraid. However, quite quickly I realised I was wasting too much time and energy on something I had no control over, so I decided to keep myself busy in the coming months.

Every morning I woke to the sound of seagulls calling outside my bedroom window. I would listen to the sound of the waves crashing on the beach and this calmed my mind. I enjoyed watching the gulls glide gracefully through the sky, and observed the sea sparkling in the distance.

I completed my coursework in the afternoons while my daughter was napping, and flew back to London twice to complete the final modules of the course. Then I started seeing clients for free, to get some experience. I joined mother and toddler groups, and I went for long walks on the beach to soak in the sea air and blow away the cobwebs from the past.

I was so determined that I was going to make positive changes in my life. I journaled every night, I listened to hypnosis recordings, and I worked on my mindset. I attended a holistic course on the Law of Attraction and kept my mind occupied. Some days I felt weepy and craved my old life and friendships, and other days I was distracted by studying. Bit by bit I was adjusting. Every day brought new opportunities and walks on the beach that blew away the old cobwebs of the past.

Eight months later, I got my own home – and it felt amazing. It was a brand-new start, and something I had visualised every night. I had my own space again, with a garden for my daughter. I started to build my business and won several awards. Slowly but surely, I began to find my way again. I felt like I was re-blossoming. I met a new and wonderful man, and my life started to slot back into place again.

And then my life was forced to take a sharp turn in another direction, when a few years later in my early 40s, I discovered that I had gone into an early menopause. My emotions had been all over the place, and I went for a series of blood tests over six months. I found myself bursting into tears over little things like a TV advert that previously would have had no effect on me, and I felt constantly on edge. I experienced hot flushes, headaches, achy bones, and extreme tiredness. I didn't feel like me at all. I suddenly felt older and an anomaly from the other – younger – school mums who were also taking their four-year-old children to primary school.

I was put on HRT, and during the first weeks of medication I experienced what felt like a panic attack walking into a shopping centre. Later, that same feeling came back when I was out driving my car. *What was going on?* I didn't know what was happening to me. I didn't feel like me any more. I had rebuilt my life, and now this was happening. It didn't seem fair!

I was so frustrated and did not feel attractive any more. My self-worth took a real nosedive. I was then referred to a specialist who adjusted my dosage of HRT, and this made all the difference. I started to feel like me again. As the months went by, I started to increase my energy levels by joining the local gym and going to Zumba and aqua fit lessons. I started to feel better mentally. Light began to come back into my life again, and I started to experience joy and contentment. I felt stronger inside.

The experience taught me more about the human mind and how we are constantly changing and growing. I hadn't collapsed. I was able to take one heavy foot in front of the other and take steps into the future without having a clue what it would hold. I was able to make the leap, and so can you.

I am choosing to enjoy my life with my daughter. As I type this now, I am sitting in my home looking out at my garden full of trees coming into blossom. The sun is shining and the sky is a clear blue. I can hear the birds singing and I can see the branches of my weeping willow tree at the bottom of my garden gently floating in the breeze of the spring air. Life is good and I am strong again.

> *'The oak fought the wind and was broken, the willow bent when it must and survived.'*
> ~ Robert Jordan, *The Fires of Heaven*

# A message to my younger self...

If I could go back in time and speak to my younger self, I would want to tell her that she will not always feel the way she does. These feelings will pass. Starting from today, she needs to believe in herself. By doing this, you can defy all odds, overcome any obstacle, and rise to your greatest potential.

I would also like to tell her that she is not stuck or a failure. She will learn so much from this experience. I want to tell her to please hold onto the hope that things will change for her. Even if it feels like a tiny glimmer or chink of light being let through a curtain right now, in time the light will come flooding back in again.

Look after yourself. This is the most important gift that you can give yourself right now. Lift the blame or shame from yourself, and this will unburden your anxiety. When you start to believe in yourself, your confidence will grow and you will feel motivated to keep going, and then you will discover hidden resources and gifts inside you that you didn't know you had.

I wish I had known back then, when my world fell apart, how powerful the mind can be and how even through those dark times you can utilise your brain to manage negative thought patterns and feel calmer. I wish I had found hypnotherapy earlier, as it was so helpful for me in the months that followed my separation. It helped me to quieten down my busy brain and take me off to a lovely relaxing place, far away from the day-to-day drama. I learned how to visualise, and by envisioning the future and the life I wanted to create for myself and my daughter, I was able to keep focused.

Being able to survive everything I had been through has shown me that we are stronger and more resilient than we think we are. During difficult periods in our lives it is possible to tap into our inner resilience. It is never too late. We can evolve and adapt through our life experiences. Through my work with clients, I am constantly amazed at how resourceful we as humans are at overcoming adversity.

If I could get through some difficult times in my life and adapt to changes in my body, I know you can, too.

I now feel excited about my future and honoured to have shared some of my story with you. I am determined to use my knowledge to help others find their path in life.

I am a strong, tenacious, determined woman, who refuses to quit, no matter what comes my way. I look forward to discovering the next chapter in my life. I now know I have the strength within me, and can use the tools I have to help me.

*I am The Girl Who Refused to Quit.*

## Dedication

To Daisy my little bundle of energy remember to always be you and keep laughing. To Bryan and my mum for supporting me always.

## About the author

Judith, who lives in Bangor in N.Ireland has been described as having a calm healing energy.

When she is not running her hypnotherapy business helping clients overcoming anxieties and fears and moving on with their lives, Judith can be found cooking and walking on the beach. She is a single parent and used hypnotherapy to transform her life.

She writes hypnosis recordings that have been described as magical healing stories. She is currently writing her first solo book.

Judith's mission is to heal women who are feeling stuck and want to move on with their lives.

## Contact

Email: info@judithwardhypnotherapy.co.uk
Website: www.judithwardhypnotherapy.co.uk
Facebook: /judithwardhypnotherapy
Linkedin: /judithwardhypnotherapy

# Chasing Freedom

## Shanna Rose

I sat in my doctor's office, feeling apprehensive, before she went on to explain that visual migraines were the cause of the temporary loss of vision I kept experiencing. It was a huge relief to know that it wasn't due to anything more serious. Looking back through my notes, she could see I'd seen another doctor earlier that year because I was suffering from poor concentration, lethargy, and all over body aches, amongst other things. I'd been sent for various blood tests which had all come back clear.

She looked up from my notes and asked me how I was feeling… really feeling. Was I stressed? I burst into floods of tears out of nowhere, refused the offer of medication, but walked out with a note signing me off work for two weeks, due to stress.

Driving home, I began thinking about this opportunity of two weeks off work. I hadn't had two full weeks off work in years, never mind whilst my children were attending school five days a week. I could get loads done with this time to myself! Yes, being signed off with stress was rubbish, but I could still make the most of a shit situation by using the time productively.

Once back home, I made myself a brew, sat on the sofa, and gave some more thought to what my doctor had said about the visual migraines and the blood tests that had come back clear. I'd felt myself burning out for a while now, but instead of resting I'd continued to push myself even more, believing that the harder I worked, the sooner I would get to slow down.

I didn't have any GCSEs to my name, never mind a degree, like most people I've ever worked alongside. So ever since my first job at 16, I would always push myself above and beyond, constantly striving for more. I always felt I had something to prove.

I was good at my job and damn proud to have worked my way up from the bottom and achieved what I had throughout my career. But I was always taking on more responsibility, spinning more and more plates. And now I felt like I couldn't escape from people's expectations of me. I'd also set up a side business, as part of my escape plan to leave the corporate world, but working full time and raising two children meant I often found myself working on my side business till the early hours.

I was tired, for sure. I'd also spoken to my dad recently for the first time since I'd turned twelve. He had got hold of my mum's telephone number through a friend of a friend, and curiosity about what he'd wanted to say had made me return his call. *Would the decades have changed him and had him wanting to make peace with his past?* It turned out that, no, it hadn't. I never got an apology, but what I did get were the flashbacks from hearing his voice again, of memories I hadn't realised were there.

I decided that some time to slow down would probably

be for the best. It wasn't just affecting me mentally, but physically too, and I'd be no good to my boys the way I was going at this rate. I needed to put my health first. So, I made the decision to take the doctor's advice and take two weeks off. Properly off, too.

Stopping for the first time in years saw me mentally crashing hard, and I was signed off for a few weeks more. This time, I accepted some medication. The doctor explained to me that if I had a broken leg, I'd have a cast on to support it whilst it healed, so I should think of the medicine like a temporary support for my mind whilst I climbed my way out.

The early days of the breakdown remain a bit of a blur. What I do remember is my partner taking the boys to school and picking them up again. I remember being laid in bed thinking what a failure and a shit mum I was. I had pushed myself all my life, overcome trauma, and had climbed the corporate career ladder... to now what? To be unable to do anything? All that fucking hard work and pain over the years had led to this? What a joke I was. In fact, not even a joke; it wasn't even funny, it was pathetic. I felt pathetic.

As the weeks passed, I began coming up for air. I'd moved to the sofa from the bed, was bathing again, and had started leaving the house to do the school run. I would stay in the car whilst I dropped my boys off, then drive straight home and continue to make my way through the housework which had recently been ignored, whilst psyching myself up to put on my happy face once again in time to pick them up. And repeat each day. Things I once used to do without thinking were all now giant steps in my healing.

After a few weeks of building myself up again, I decided it was time to figure my way out of this dark place. I had overcome so much in my life, and refused to play victim once again and remain at rock bottom. I'd had years of practice of self-healing, learning to love myself, and had become extremely self-aware. It was time to put all I had learnt over the years into action. But before I could think of what to do to get out of the darkness, I first needed to look inward and give some thought to understanding how I had got here in the first place.

There was only one other time in my life, besides this breakdown, when I can remember feeling like my world had suddenly collapsed on me, as though my life had been turned upside down and I didn't know the way out.

I was sitting in a cell at the police station – and not for the first time. I used to run away from home a lot as a kid, and then from my foster home when I first entered the care system. As I was under sixteen, I'd be reported missing to the police and they'd either take me back home or to my foster place, depending on where I was living at the time. If I resisted, they'd shove me in the back of their van and take me to the police station, where I would sit in a cell for a few hours before someone came to collect me – usually my mum.

This one time I was in the cell and the usual few hours had passed, but there was no sign of my mum. The next morning came and there was still no sign of her. Lying on the hard mattress staring at the ceiling, I had nothing else to do but think. What had my life come to?

As a child, I'd had a very strict religious upbringing, having to prove myself worthy of God's love every day. I wasn't allowed the middle page poster from my *Smash Hits* music magazine on my bedside table, as it was a form of idolisation, and the only person I should be idolising was God.

We would never celebrate or join others in celebrating Christmas, birthdays, or any other traditional celebratory periods. Throughout primary school, I was that girl telling all the other kids that Santa wasn't real. For religious education lessons, the teachers had been instructed to remove me from class, and I would sit alone in the cloakroom reading my book until the lesson finished. It was the same with any other lessons or activities related to religion – Christmas, Easter, or even Mother's Day – throughout school. During assembly, when everyone gathered in the hall each week and sang songs, some of which were hymns – yep, you guessed it, I'd be sat back in the cloakroom with just the usual coats and hanging PE kits for company, reading my book once again.

To say I felt lonely and like I didn't fit in would be an understatement. I'd just bury my head in my book and my mind would be whisked away on different amazing adventures.

I would continue to find escape in reading books at home, too. My dad used to hit me, and I don't just mean a smack on the hand. Sometimes he would take his leather-soled slipper off and hit me repeatedly with it. I'd be curled up in a ball in a corner, shielding my face, and it wouldn't take long until I could no longer scream out because I was hyperventilating that much. I'd then be carried to the bathroom and cold wet flannels would be laid over my red, throbbing skin whilst I lay sobbing on the floor. The bathmat was orange – a peachy orange – and I'd look at the threads hanging over the edge, all sticking out in different directions, and try to count them. If a book wasn't in my hands, I became good at finding other means of escape.

It wasn't just physical abuse, either. I remember being reminded to feed my rabbit, Pipkin, but he wasn't in his cage or run. He must have escaped somehow. It took me a while of searching everywhere before my dad, laughing, let me in on the joke; he'd given my rabbit away. Then one day he returned from work with a surprise for me and my brother – a kitten each. I was so happy I had something else to love and care for even though I still missed Pipkin. It didn't last long, though. He stood on my kitten's head and killed her in front of me.

I'd try so hard to act in a way I would fit in and be liked. That, combined with having to prove how worthy of God's love I was, was definitely a recipe for a childhood – and later years – spent constantly betraying myself in order to win the love and affection of others.

I was twelve years old when my mum and dad separated. Me and my brother moved to another city with my mum, and that's where I started secondary school.

I remember getting caught a couple of times with the top button undone on my school shirt, so I was given one thousand lines to do as punishment. I then got caught with it unbuttoned again that same week, so I was given a detention.

I felt so angry at the system, especially after a childhood spent walking around on eggshells trying not to get hit. A childhood spent feeling trapped in a religion I hated. Being punished for having a shirt button undone definitely triggered me. I'd spent my childhood respecting authority figures – my dad, teachers, even a 'god' – and look where that had got me. No-one had fucking helped that little girl sobbing on the bathmat when she needed it most.

I had learnt my lesson the hard way and decided no-one would get respect from me any more purely because they were in a position of authority. The more people tried to make me conform, the more I would rebel.

Now thirteen years old, I realised I couldn't be forced to do anything I didn't want to do. The next time I got given a detention, I walked out of the school. My mum grounded me, so I walked out of the house anyway. I had lost all respect for authority figures and I felt free for the first time ever. No teachers to boss me around, no parents, no God to answer to. Just me and the older friends I'd made, all hanging out together.

Going back to the police cell where I was sitting, and fast forward a few more hours and there was still no sign of my mum. I'd certainly had plenty of time to think about not only my past but my future, too. I realised I couldn't carry on like this. I was directing all of my energy into finally feeling free and doing whatever the hell I wanted, whereas in reality I'd got myself expelled from school, had been using my new-found freedom to hang out in bus shelters, and was currently locked in a police cell. This freedom I'd been chasing certainly sucked in reality.

I knew I needed to sort my life out somehow and face my past. I decided that when my mum finally came to get me, I would tell her how sorry I was and ask how to get help.

When the cell door finally opened, I felt relieved. Maybe

I could make an effort and have a fresh start? I walked to the reception area to find it wasn't my mum waiting for me. It was a social worker; one I hadn't met before. So that's what took so long. It was because my mum wasn't coming for me.

I was told I was being taken to a children's home in another city, and that my stuff was in a bin bag inside the car. That moment, right then, was the first time that I felt my world collapse in on me. It was like the floor had been taken out from under me and I was free-falling.

Sitting in the back of the social worker's car, my head leaning against the window, I took back everything I'd agreed with myself in the police cell. Fuck everyone once again! Fuck the world! And to think I had been going to ask for help to try to sort my life out. Now I was being sent away with just a bin bag.

I stayed in that children's home for weeks before being moved to an even bigger eight-bedroomed one – home to other young people who'd had troubled upbringings or had been through adversity of some kind. For the first time in my life, I actually felt like I fitted in. I'd found people just like me. I also found drugs, and spent the next couple of years continuing my self-destructive behaviour, feeling like I was sticking two fingers up to the world.

I was fifteen years old when I was told I couldn't stay there much longer. No-one stayed beyond sixteen, as bedrooms were then given to other children in need. I knew this was my chance. I decided to move away to another city, cut all contact with the 'friends' I was self-destructing with, and start afresh.

I found a flat, and at just fifteen years old I was living alone. No-one to tell me what to do, no-one to give me a curfew for the first time in my life, and no-one to punish me for leaving the top button undone on my shirt. I found a job where I could gain a qualification, and was determined to prove wrong everyone I'd encountered over the years. I'd prove my dad wrong, my teachers, social workers, and even my old friends. I would show them they were all wrong about me. I would make something of my life.

Fast forward a few years, and I entered a relationship with someone who would eventually start to push me around and be violent. I'd want to leave him, but then he would get upset with himself for hitting me, so I'd end up staying and comforting him instead. I had grown up being hit for years as a child, so it was normal, but my dad had never apologised or got upset. Maybe this was what true love looked like?

I finally made my escape and ended the relationship, and that was when my self-healing journey truly took off. I spent the following years growing so much love for myself.

But I was still constantly striving for more. I would never stay satisfied with any success and was always seeking the next challenge to overcome. It was exhilarating achieving all the things, and had become addictive. It made me feel good about myself, as though I was valuable and worth something, like I was no longer that unloved or unwanted little girl.

Since just before my sixteenth birthday I had tried so hard to do the opposite of what I'd done as a young teen when I went off the rails. I thought trying to fit in to what society dictated would be the way to prove everyone wrong, how to make something of my life, but now I felt trapped in a life of my own creation. With just my income alone to rely on, I'd wonder how I would ever escape the corporate world, be my own boss, and finally live a life that fulfilled me and was staying true to myself.

When my salary then dropped thousands of pounds due to a lack of funding, but the job role and my responsibilities remained the same, it hit me hard – and not just financially. My dad had got back in touch and along came the flashbacks. I had been burning myself out at work taking on more and more responsibility, whilst also working on my side business. I crashed big time.

Yes, I'd had an amazing self-love journey over the last few years, had two amazing children, a good career, and a beautiful house, but I was still trying to prove something by fitting into someone else's mould of me. When fitting in means truly suppressing who we are, we miss the opportunity to live an extraordinary life on our own terms.

Looking deeply inward about what had caused my breakdown and the why behind me burning myself out, I had a sudden realisation: I didn't need to prove anything at all. I never have. I am already enough, and I always have been.

The freedom I had been chasing all my life was never another achievement away. It was never an external thing. Freedom was a feeling that had been inside of me all along just waiting to be uncovered.

I am free.

## *A message to my younger self...*

If I could go back in time and speak to my younger self, I would give that little girl such a big hug and tell her I love her so much. She is amazing just as she is, and one day will discover just how beautiful and fun life can be.

I wish I had known that we are each enough just as we are. No-one should strive to feel valid or worthy. We are already all of these things.

Being able to survive everything I have been through has shown me that we are not our pasts. Yesterday doesn't matter. We get to decide who we show up as every day, and have the power to create a life we love, no matter what our history.

I now feel free.

I am still wearing the top button undone on my shirts.

*I am The Girl Who Refused to Quit.*

## Dedication

To the woman who has struggled to love herself, or who has ever wondered why she wasn't enough. You can rewrite your story too. You are enough exactly as you are right now and always have been.

## About the author

Shanna lives with her family in the countryside of North Yorkshire, England. She has been described as fun loving, inspirational and with a huge passion for helping others. She is also a proud Mum of two boys that are growing far too quick.

Her mission is to show people that their pasts do not define their future and that we are all full of unlimited potential. Through her coaching business she helps women come home to themselves, find their inner compass and turn their struggles into superpowers so they can live a life they love.

When she's not coaching clients she can often be found where there is a view or pursuing her love of live music. A massive nature lover she credits her love of the outdoors with her keeping her sanity over the years.

## Contact

www.shanna-rose.com
Instagram: @_shanna_rose_
Facebook: Shanna Rose

# Ready to Fly
## *Nicola Creen*

From as far back as I can remember, I was always bullied as a child. A combination of emotional and physical bullying, name-calling, getting beaten up became normal. I remember thinking, *What is wrong with me? Why am I always the target?* I would cry myself to sleep every night, wondering what I could do to fit in, and how I could avoid the same thing happening the following day.

I know now it was because of my looks and ambition. Fast forward to the age of seventeen, after suffering more bullying through primary and high school. As the years went on, it seemed to get worse, and I eventually had a nervous breakdown. I refused to take any medication, and that was the beginning of my journey into wellness.

I swore to myself I would never let things get that bad again. I could see my bubbly personality starting to shine through again, and by the age of twenty-one, I had built a great life for myself.

I secured a management position at the local airport hotel, I was engaged to be married, and life was sweet. But that wasn't to last long. One night at work, during night shift, I started suffering horrendous pains in my stomach. I put it down to period cramps, but they kept getting stronger and stronger. A member of staff got me some painkillers, but it continued to get worse!

The next morning, I remember having to crawl up the stairs to my flat. I was in so much pain, it was unbearable! My dad came and phoned the doctor, who sent an ambulance to rush me to hospital straight away. I ended up having emergency lifesaving surgery where I lost seven pints of blood, one of my fallopian tubes, and my first baby. I'll never forget how upset my family looked after the surgery. The surgeon said that another ten minutes and I would have also lost my life.

Looking back, I know I was in so much shock that I pushed all that pain deep down and carried on. I felt grateful to be alive, but I never allowed myself to grieve for the baby I'd lost. Things didn't work out in my relationship, so I packed up and moved from Scotland to Manchester, once again rebuilding my life and doing well for myself career-wise.

At the age of twenty-nine, by a sheer medical miracle, I was a mum! By that point, I had done some modelling, but because of the continued bullying and unwanted attention, I didn't pursue it seriously. So, when I got asked to take part in a photoshoot at the age of twenty-nine, I jumped at the chance!

I remember some naysayers saying, 'You'll never get anywhere, you're too old,' etc, but I ended up crying happy tears when I got the phone call to say that not only had I been recognised, but I'd been selected to be a finalist in London's west end for Top Model UK. I could not believe it! The news made the headlines, and I was headhunted to take part in a Scottish beauty pageant.

At first, the thought of being in an environment

surrounded by bitchy girls filled me with horror, and I refused to take part on a number of occasions. Despite my reservations, the event photographer insisted I give it some thought, and told me I'd be a perfect candidate as they wanted someone who was beautiful not just on the outside, but inside, too. Eventually, I took his advice and decided to go for it. After all, what did I have to lose? I recall thinking it would be something my son could be proud of.

As the weeks flew by in the build up to the event, sure enough the bitchy comments started, and certain finalists already had themselves down as being the winner. I honestly never thought for a minute that I could win; after all, I was around ten years older than the other finalists. But I remember thinking that when I got out on the stage, I would hold my head high. There were three rounds in the competition. The first was tartan wear, and I managed to secure a one-off piece made by a designer in London, which was unreal! The second round was swimwear, and the final round evening wear, for which I wore a beautiful blue princess-style dress from America. We also had to write our own speech about why we should win.

It was my mum's 50th birthday that night, and the whole family was there to support me in the biggest ballroom in Glasgow's Crown Plaza Hotel. The event organiser instructed me to go first and I could see the other finalists giving me nasty looks as I unpacked my dresses.

I'll never forget hearing the host announce, 'Ladies and gentlemen, please welcome Nicola Creen onto the stage.' I could hear everyone clapping, but instead of feeling proud, I felt mortified. I should have been ready to walk down the catwalk, but I was struggling to put on my dress, as it was so heavy. Every other finalist stood there watching me struggle, not one of them offered to help! I remember wondering how they could do that; it was like they were enjoying it! If the roles had been reversed, I would have been the first person to offer help! Thankfully, I got a member of the hotel staff to help me, and off I went.

When it came to everyone's turn to read their speech, one of the girls who had said throughout she would win, actually ran off the stage crying. It seemed as though nerves had got the better of her. My turn came and, still believing I had no chance of winning, I let the words flow passionately from my heart. I told the audience that if I won, I would always use this experience as a platform to help as many people as I could. I finished by telling them not to allow the naysayers to stop them pursuing their dreams, and to never give up on themselves. I had given it my all, and left the stage feeling proud that I had used my voice to help empower others.

We were told to wait backstage as the judges decided who the top five would be, before announcing the overall winner. Sitting quietly backstage, I started to take off my jewellery, genuinely believing that the night, and the experience, were over for me.

We were instructed to stand in line as they announced the top five, and I wished everyone good luck, never thinking for a minute that my name would be called. There was a big build-up and drum roll, and I'll never forget the moment the host announced the first top five finalist as… Nicola Creen! I was absolutely gobsmacked and completely overwhelmed with emotion and happy tears.

Onto the stage (in shock!) I went with the other four

finalists. Then, after yet another big build-up, we heard, 'The winner is… Nicola Creen!' Me? OMG! My legs collapsed from shock as I fell to the floor on my knees, head in my hands, sobbing! *Was this really happening? How could I be the winner, against all the odds?* To this day, I still have to pinch myself!

We celebrated my win and my mum's birthday for the rest of the weekend. Still smiling in my happy bubble, I logged onto Facebook for the first time on the Monday to find I had been bombarded with loads of congratulations messages. And then… in a single moment, everything changed! One of the finalists had found a really old picture of me from years before, not long after I'd given birth to my son. I looked heavy, tired, and pale, and she had shamelessly shared that image across the whole of social media, along with the sarcastic message, *I didn't win, but here's your winner!*

What was going on? My whole stomach turned and the tears flowed as I read the horrible comments about me, from people that didn't even know me. What should have been the happiest time had become absolutely horrendous. I felt so hurt. I cried for hours.

After taking some time to get over the hurt, I decided to dig deep for some determination so that I could stay true to my word. I started my own academy for girls who wanted to shine in a safe environment – a place where I could instil confidence from within, and teach them how to overcome bullying, etc. Once again, career-wise everything was amazing.

Unfortunately, though, my happiness didn't last long. After being swept off my feet and thinking I'd met the man of my dreams, I ended up in an abusive relationship which resulted in me becoming homeless and pregnant at the same time. I'd already been through so much, but this was my ultimate rock bottom. He tried to destroy my life and my career, and I was forced to use all the strength I had to not only survive but thrive, for the sake of my son and unborn daughter.

I'll be honest, there were many nights when I felt like giving up, crying myself to sleep, wondering how was I going to bring my unborn child into the world as a single mum who had lost everything. One of my best friends slept on her couch and allowed me, my unborn baby, and my son, to have her bed while I desperately tried to figure out what I was going to do. Slowly, I started getting my strength back and survival mode kicked in. I took really good care of myself; I began meditating, and visualised how my life could look if I just pulled the strength together to get through this period.

I was around five months pregnant when I got the news that I had secured a flat for the three of us. I'd never had my own council flat before, but it felt like a lottery win! A little haven where we could be safe, and I could start to rebuild my life again. My ex-partner had convinced me that nobody would want me and that my career was over, but I was determined to survive.

I racked my brains about what I could do. When my son was at nursery school one day a week, I went to the library as I didn't have the internet connected at home. And it was on one of these library visits that I had a light bulb moment. Many years before, I'd had my own local radio show called *The Feel-Good Friday Show,* which ran for three years. That was it! I had the most overwhelming feeling to find a way to get back into radio.

I had tried on numerous occasions to get into the BBC without any success, so this time I thought I'd do some research. I Googled the head of the BBC Radio Scotland at that time and found out it was Jeff Zycinski. I remember looking for him on Facebook and wondering whether or not I should message him. *Again, what did I have to lose?* I was shaking with nerves and anticipation as I sent him a message on Messenger, explaining that I had radio presenting experience and would be grateful for any advice.

I nearly gave birth on the chair when I saw him typing back straight away! He told me to meet him at the BBC on Monday at 2pm. I couldn't believe it! I was overwhelmed with excitement that after all these years I was being invited into the BBC.

That Monday, wearing my best dress and my most prized Louboutin shoes, I found myself sitting in front of the man himself. I was honest with him about the fact that I was pregnant, and we agreed to stay in touch. I didn't think anything of it; I had convinced myself that once again, I had been unsuccessful in getting into the BBC.

As soon as we moved into our flat, the horrendous morning sickness stopped, and I found I had a whole new lease of life! I started to see light at the end of the tunnel and knew that this experience was not going to define me. I was not going to let that man ruin my life. I made the flat into our beautiful little safe haven, and we loved it. We had a balcony with the most beautiful views, and I felt as though this was another chance to start again. I was determined to give my babies the best life possible.

As soon as my ex got wind that his ploy to destroy me wasn't working, he stalked me, followed me, and threatened me. I had to get the police involved, and the stress started taking its toll on my unborn child. Every night I would cry myself to sleep again, terrified that I might lose her. Her movements were very irregular, and I had to be admitted to hospital every other day, wired up to heart monitors to make sure she was ok.

I remember looking around the ward; other women had their men there to support them, and there was me with my son holding my hand through it all. He should have been playing with his friends during the summer, but was with me in hospital instead. Eventually, the doctors decided that the stress was too much, and I was to be induced.

My son wen to stay with his dad, who has been amazing throughout, and my mum and my Nan were with me as I started the labour process, which was to last for a terrifying thirty-three hours. When the doctor decided that I would have to go for a C-section because I was so exhausted and the baby in too much distress, I asked to give one last push. Gathering every bit of the strength I had left, I pushed… and there she was. My little miracle was born. As she was still unwell, she had to go into the special care unit for a few days to be monitored. It killed me not having her with me, but I was so relieved that she had been born and that the nightmare of a pregnancy was over.

The days and nights that followed were so difficult – doing everything on my own, night feeds, etc – but I was consumed with love for both my children, and knew I was going to create a great life for them.

A year later, I was out doing a food shop with the two kids, when I received a message from Jeff asking me if I wanted to present my own show on the BBC on a Friday night? I could apparently pick my favourite songs and chat to our national listeners. OMG! I was in tears of pure joy. Finally, I had achieved success, after the heartache of everything. After thinking my life was over, I was being given a lifeline. I will be forever grateful to Jeff for believing in me and giving me an amazing opportunity. Five years on, I still contribute on the BBC, and that has led to so many other amazing opportunities.

Now my kids look at the media articles and testimonials and tell me how proud they are of me, which is just the best feeling in the world! Both my kids bring me so much joy. After years of thinking I wouldn't be able to have children, I feel so very grateful every day that I get to be a mum.

*How is life now?* Well, let's just say I have gained an abundance of wisdom and resilience, plus so much more. I am now a successful life/business coach, BBC broadcaster, lecturer, international keynote inspirational speaker, and by autumn I will be a published author. I have used all my pain to help inspire, empower, and encourage people from all over the world, and show that if I can go through all that and come out the other end, they can get through anything, too. I want everyone reading about me to feel inspired and never to give up on themselves or their dreams.

I've experienced so many ups and downs. People I thought were friends have taken advantage; potential love interests have painted the picture of being yet another knight in shining armour, only to let me down again.

When I look back on it all now, though, I would not change a single thing. My work has been featured globally and I'm proud that I turned all that pain into something positive. I've saved the lives of suicidal clients and worked in schools, encouraging our young to never give up on their dreams of starting their own business. I have countless lifesaving and life-changing testimonials which make every bit of pain and suffering worth it all! I've achieved more than I could ever have dreamed of.

The whole journey has shaped me into who I am today. I believe I was meant to go through all of this to become a beacon of light and strength to so many out there who are suffering. And there's not a day goes by that I don't feel immense gratitude for my life, my miracle babies, and the real, genuine people in my life that were there for me.

As I write this, we are in the midst of a global COVID-19 pandemic, and there are so many more stories to tell.

I wouldn't change a thing, and if you get anything from reading this, I want you to know that there's absolutely so much strength inside of you that you don't even realise it. If I can get through everything I have, you can, too!

Please, never give up on yourself. Life is a beautiful gift, and I promise you that better days do come. Stars don't shine without the darkness, so don't let your hard times make you feel shame or embarrassment.

I feel like this is just the beginning and I know that this has all happened for a reason. I'm ready to fly.

## A message to my younger self...

If I could go back in time and speak to my younger self, I would tell her that there's going to be so many painful moments in her life, but to know that she has absolutely everything inside of her to get through them.

I have massive appreciation for everything that's happened in my life until this point – even the bad, as I know without all that pain and the many lessons I've learned, I wouldn't be half the woman I am today. I'm so much more resilient, stronger, grateful, and happier as a result.

I would tell her that these painful times will make her stronger and much happier in the long run. That without the darkness the stars wouldn't shine, and that's exactly how her life is going to pan out. There's going to be a lot of darkness, but that is exactly what's going to make her shine brighter than ever and go on to inspire so many people from all over the world.

I wish I had known back then just how strong I was going to become and not made decisions out of fear or lack of self-worth, that I was more than enough and didn't need any validation from anyone to feel that. I would tell her to not look for love in the wrong places and to love herself first and foremost.

Being able to survive everything I have has shown me that I can overcome anything, that nothing and nobody will get in my way and, more importantly, that I am an example to my beautiful children and amazing clients that you really can live the life of your dreams against all the odds.

I now feel more empowered than ever before. I feel free. Free of the opinion of others. Free from my past. More grateful and excited about the future than ever before.

I am walking proof that you can go through the toughest of times, get knocked down time and time again, and come out the other end... stronger... happier... and healthier.

*I am The Girl Who Refused to Quit.*

## Dedication

To my babies. My whole world. My inspiration. You are why I show up relentlessly every day and my reason for being the girl who refused to quit.

## About the author

Nicola who lives near Glasgow in Scotland has been described as an "angel on earth with the heart of a lion, unbelievable strength and a huge passion for helping people".

When she's not speaking on stage, writing, coaching, featuring on radio, hitting the headlines and changing lives Nicola can often be found pursuing her love of travel and music but best of all enjoying quality time with her children.

She is a very proud Life/Business coach, keynote inspirational speaker and author who thrives on transforming lives and businesses on a daily basis.

Nicola's mission is to change as many lives as possible, leading by example. Teaching the tools and techniques that have not only made her and her clients survive but thrive against all the odds.

## Contact

E mail: nicolacreenacademy@gmail.com

# Dance For Your Heart
## Natalie Kyne-Dinsdale

### Becoming Mummy

February 2013 began with sadness, when my funny and caring Grandad sadly passed away. He would often take me to dance class if my parents weren't able to. He would often come to watch me in dance performances. When I was just ten years old, he suddenly had a stroke and his world changed drastically. He had to re-learn how to talk, walk, and drive, but he was determined – some would say stubborn – enough to do so, and we are all grateful that he was. Subconsciously, I have been using him as my role model for years, reminding me not to give up when things get tough.

That same month was also when my husband David and I found out that we were expecting our first child. We were both so happy and couldn't wait to tell our parents and, more importantly, my Nan, who right then needed something to look forward to. As we expected, they were all excited and emotional.

For as long as I can remember, I have been very passionate about alternative therapies and love how our bodies are stronger than we sometimes give them credit for. I knew, before my pregnancy, that I wanted a natural water birth. We went to a hypnobirthing course and I am so pleased that my husband understands visualisation and meditation, as he uses it for his astounding performances for his ice-skating competitions, so he was able to encourage me and join in with the sessions really well.

It was no surprise, however, that a number of friends I mentioned it to would dismiss the amazing power of our mind and would tell me, 'It will still hurt!' Without meaning to, they made me feel that I was being ridiculous. They were right, though, I had never been through labour, so how could I know? They made me doubt myself and question my mind's strength. Thankfully, a few more hypnobirthing lessons, where we worked on exercises to help manage pain, helped me to believe in the process again. Working with my breath, my body, and my own mind, I was able to reduce my anxiety.

Our son, Finn, arrived in the December 2013, and I was able to have the waterbirth I had wished for, with just a few tiny glitches. I was so grateful that I was able to reduce my anxiety. I was so calm that the midwife didn't believe my son was about to appear, and actually left the room!

I loved being a mum and felt organised and in control. I was loving life and, despite the sleepless nights, felt energetic.

## Mummy guilt

No one can prepare us for becoming parents. I'm sure you can guess that the organisation didn't last. So much worry and overwhelm, then throwing work in there just to make it a million times harder. So many things I would worry about...

*Am I doing enough for him? Am I too focused on work? Is he doing enough for his age? Am I spoiling him? Should I be taking him everywhere? Should I be leaving him at home? What if something happens to him in the care of someone else? I shouldn't be leaving him!*

Some parents make it look easy, and I always felt that I should be able to keep the house tidier. I always felt judged by the way I fed him, dressed him, and with practically anything. These were just my assumptions, and not what anyone said. I don't think there is any mum out there, especially with your first, who doesn't feel like they are getting everything wrong.

As well as being a new mum, I was working two days a week as a graphic designer and three days as an Irish Dancing teacher. For dancing, we have competitions regularly, and I have always loved being there to support our dancers. I love helping them to prepare and to ensure they feel ready to perform with confidence. Thankfully, David is always supportive of my dancing and the amount of time I spend coaching.

Before Finn was walking, I was still able to teach regularly and would take him with me. He would be in the pram while I watched the dancers, and he loved the attention from the children. However, it was not as easy to coach the dancers, because I didn't want to leave him with a random mum in a busy venue. He was my precious, gorgeous baby boy and I always struggled when I handed him over to somebody else. I also didn't want him feeling

I had abandoned him when he saw an unfamiliar face. I needed him to know I was still there for him.

When Finn was about eight months old, I started leaving him at home more to have fun with his daddy. Other times, I wouldn't go to the competition. Either way, though, I felt guilty! Guilty that I was letting my dancers down for not being there, or guilty that I was not at home with Finn and our little family.

When I did go, I absolutely loved watching our dancers and being able to offer support and guidance. I also always loved getting home for the biggest welcoming hug full of love from my little man.

## Something was changing…

Sunday mornings I would wake up, usually with Finn in bed beside me, and I was feeling exhausted and unmotivated, waking up and knowing I had to get up in front of the class to teach and be professional for the dancers. I barely had the energy to get dressed. I was starting to lose my enthusiasm and love for dance and just wanted to be home with my baby. I was ashamed to feel like this, so I kept trying to push through it.

David had been training at the ice-rink since 6am while Finn and I were dozing on and off, and I just couldn't understand why I couldn't find that motivation to keep going. I kept telling myself that I was just being lazy and that I was rubbish. I have always loved being busy and had so much energy – I used to love running in the mornings – so this feeling was just awful!

I had usually been up until 3am or later doing admin work for dancing, dropping off to sleep for a couple of seconds at the table, then carrying on. Looking back now, it wasn't the most productive way of working, but at the time I couldn't see any other solution. And I have always worked late, so didn't think much about it.

I took Finn to a number of groups to meet other children, and so that I would hopefully meet other mums, but these groups always made me feel lonely. Most of the time other parents would come along with another friend, so they generally stayed together. I stuck with the classes to try to help Finn, and we went to something every Monday, Tuesday, and Thursday, and he was at nursery every Wednesday and Friday.

We were always rushing, and my housework was stressfully mounting up. I felt like I was handing my son over to my husband and shooting out the door every Tuesday, and the same on a Thursday leaving him with my parents. I was trying to dedicate the same hours to the classes as I had before, because I didn't want to let the dancers down.

## Help!

I'll never forget the day when I got into my car after teaching a class and received a text message from one of the mums and part of it read…

*You have lost your smile!*

It felt like someone was holding my throat! Tears rolled down my face without any warning.

I allowed them to fall down my face; it was a huge release of emotions! I don't know if it was because I had just realised that I wasn't coping. For too long I had been telling myself to try harder, that I was just being lazy and ridiculous. The tears might also have been because someone had cared enough to notice.

I went onto the internet that evening and typed in 'mums struggling with work', not really expecting to find much. The results were 'Life Coaches' and 'work life balance', but my perception was that only famous people needed this. I remember thinking, *I can't go to a Life Coach, what will people think? I don't need someone planning my life!* This is funny looking back, as I have realised how valuable seeing a Life Coach was to my life and my family time.

I read more about the benefits, and I found Lucy Stanyer – not far from me – who had great reviews. I wanted to have a chat with David to gauge how he felt, but the thought of saying, out loud, that I needed this help made me feel emotional and weak, and I felt that tightness in my throat! *How should I approach it? What if he doesn't understand? Am I being stupid?*

Thankfully, he is an amazing listener, is very supportive of all my ideas, and is also my sensible head. I remember him saying, 'It would be good to chat with her about it.' He also knows I can be 'determined' – often referred to as 'stubborn', like Grandad and my dad, showing that it's definitely in the genes – so his suggestion was, 'If we are going to spend this money for the help, you need to be willing to listen to advice and do things that you may find hard.'

## *I was ready!*

I emailed Lucy straight away and we arranged to have a discovery session a couple of weeks later. Finn was 17 months old by then, and we clicked straight away over the phone as she had a daughter, not much older, and completely understood my challenges.

I vividly remember our first face-to-face session. I remember walking up a path, past a church, everything was quiet and still and, although I was nervous, I felt calm and relieved to be getting help!

We had a little bit of small talk to ease me in gently, and I had no clue what would happen a few moments later. I didn't realise how much emotion I had been bottling up. She asked me to list what I did in a typical week – hourly as much as possible – to see where I could utilise my time better.

## *My weekly schedule…*

Monday – Dance admin work | Finn's swimming lesson | Dinner | Dance admin work.

Tuesday – Baby class | Catching up on emails | Teaching (home at 10pm) Dance admin work.

Wednesday – Finn to nursery | Design work (home at 9pm) Dance admin work.

Thursday – Baby class | Catching up on emails | Teaching (home at 11pm).

Friday – Finn to nursery | Design work (home at 9pm).

Saturday – Dance work, dance rehearsals or competitions. Dance admin work.

Sunday – Teaching until 3pm, then home to my family usually with dance admin too – I hardly went to bed before 2am every day.

Reading my list, she looked at me and said, 'No wonder you are struggling. You actually don't have any time for you.'

I was going to bed so late, waking up to Finn in the night, waking up early with him, feeling vacant and empty-headed, then trying to be everywhere. 'There's no time for you, time for David and yourself, plus no time for friends. You are really burning the candle at both ends.'

When she started talking about what I was currently missing out on, tears started blurring my vision. I was trying my hardest not to let them fall, clenching my jaw so tight. I tried to stop them still when she said, 'It really sounds like you are suffering from burnout!' Then as soon as she asked, 'Are you OK?' my tears just fell like heavy weights, relieving the pressure that I had unknowingly been hiding.

I had never heard of this as a condition before, but as soon as Lucy said the word 'burnout', I felt a strange emotional release, that someone actually understood me and why I was feeling this way.

I was feeling exhausted, empty, distant from my work, overwhelmed, and unable to cope with the demands of being a mum plus a businesswoman. I was feeling particularly lonely at that time, as I wasn't often meeting up with my friends from my pre-baby days. Their children were either not the same age, they didn't have children, or they didn't live close by, because we had moved over twenty miles away. And sadly, I hadn't made any new mummy friends at the groups either.

I couldn't explain to anyone how I was feeling as I hadn't really noticed it happening, but even after acknowledging it, I was worried to talk about it. I didn't want people to judge me and to think that I was making more of it than it needed to be. They might just think it was me being rubbish at time management.

I did start making more time to meet up with friends. When I met up with one friend over dinner, she asked how I had been, and I excitedly told her about my life coach sessions. She didn't mean to, but her reply was frustrating and seemed to just brush over my feelings when she said, 'Isn't it just common sense?' Her response made me feel pathetic, so I didn't elaborate and just left it at that.

Yes, it absolutely is common sense, and a lot of family and friends would say I was doing too much. But it was easy to state the obvious. I needed guidance and someone to show me a way out of the busy and exhausting cycle.

I have friends and family who have suffered with mental health issues and I have seen how it has had a huge impact on their lives, sometimes requiring medication to help relieve the symptoms. I have always felt that mentioning my symptoms would make them think I was searching for attention, and I didn't want to take away from the help they needed.

When I started writing this story, other people's opinions worried me and I questioned myself numerous times, but I have also realised that this story is not about me but about who else it can help. Although burnout isn't a diagnosable psychological disorder, it should still be taken seriously and be more recognised.

This was also the first time I had realised that it is not selfish to care about ourselves; it is absolutely necessary.

## Guidance

In one of our meetings, we assessed how much time I was spending on admin, planning, and teaching for dancing, which was causing me to spend so much time away from the family and for very little income. It just about covered the cost of the hall hire and fuel, but it also caused a lot of stress, pain, and anxiety when it came to shows and competitions.

Lucy suggested taking teaching out of the plan, and we considered how much time I would then have back with my family. This sounded fantastic! 'Yes, this makes so much sense,' I agreed. 'I won't have to be out of the house for so long!'

I left Lucy's office and as I was driving, on my way to my design job, my heart was way stronger than my head and it interrupted any logical thoughts. My eyes were initially a little watery, then quite quickly I couldn't stop the tears falling. Thoughts in my head were all over the place... *I can't give it up! I love teaching! I have worked so hard to get to here! I have put my heart and soul into exams, competitions, and building up my classes. I can't!*

I went back to Lucy the following week and explained my muddled thoughts. I felt like we were back to square one, but Lucy reminded me that this was part of the process!

She suggested instead about reducing the design work, so I asked for one day only at the freelance job. This meant that I could use one of the two days that Finn was at nursery to work on my business, rather than doing it all at night. This meant that I still had freelance money coming in – even though it was reduced – but it also meant I was able to collect Finn from nursery one of the days. 'This will be amazing!'

Finn used to go into nursery crying then, after a while, looking at me with such sad eyes, or trying to hold back and hang onto my leg. After a while, he had become more used to the situation and would wander off to play with a member of staff, knowing that he just had to put up with it. But I always felt like his heart was breaking as much as mine! And I was never able to collect him either, as my work was in London and I finished after 7.30pm.

Although the dancing was unsociable hours, Finn was with people he loved – either his grandparents or his daddy – and we both felt happier. My change of freelance hours meant he did still go into nursery, but I was now able to pick him up on the Wednesday, and I loved seeing his happy face come running over to me. I had been missing out on this for over a year and we both needed this!

## *Positive mind!*

After a few more sessions with Lucy, she had given me tools to use to help me plan better. This resulted in me making more time for self-care, and I was using meditations, hypnobirthing music and breathing, and Emotional Freedom Technique tapping therapy to help me. All of this positive energy had re-ignited my passion for my dance and fitness.

Over the following months, I got straight to work with preparing for workshops, which included positive mindset work, fitness for dance, and helping to prepare the dancers and their parents for competitions. I started to have time to step back and notice that our dancing mums were as frazzled as me, and they needed me to help them with advice. Show ideas started to flow better, my whole attitude towards dancing was making me feel energetic again, and my motivation had been re-ignited.

Since becoming a mum, I had forgotten everything that I had to offer as a dancing coach. Apart from being an Irish Dancing Teacher (TCRG), I am also a fully trained fitness instructor, personal trainer and nutritionist. I had studied hard and sat the exams for these, so that I could help my dancers as much as possible. Somewhere, in my parenthood journey, I had stopped using my skills and this affected my teaching, as I had started to doubt myself and lost my confidence. I had lost my self-worth and self-belief, as well as my smile. And everything had become worse through being so busy and lack of preparation.

Now that I was starting to feel my passion, motivation, and energy coming back, I was loving going to class and seeing all of my fabulous students eager to learn. I was back! I was here for my family, my dancers, and myself!

## COVID-19 and lockdown!

In the past four years, so much has happened to make me question my ability, test my strength, and cause many tears, but I have managed to find ways to help. As I am writing this story, the whole world is in Lockdown. We have the awful COVID-19 (Coronavirus Disease 2019) spreading around the world at a fast rate and proving deadly to so many.

I have a few plates spinning – not wanting to turn work away – so I am a little nervous about burnout creeping up on me again. However, I am so grateful that I can teach over video calls, I can design virtually, and I can get my health and wellness products to my customers.

This time has made me reassess my workload, reminding me that life can be so cruel and quickly taken away. I am also more mindful of work boundaries, and plan better to enjoy time with my family.

Mindfulness within the dancing world, especially around the dancers' competitions, is so important to me and I will always teach dance to promote this. I always aim to build the children up to have strong self-esteem, to realise their self-worth, to love dance, and to be kind on and off-stage!

Realising my own self-worth has enabled me to truly smile once again!


## Two Worlds, One Heart
*By Natalie Kyne-Dinsdale*

I'm a teacher of dance and soon to be mummy,
I love how my baby dances around in my tummy;
I am here for my dancers when you need me the most,
I want you to know that I'll reply to your post!

I'm a teacher of dance and my baby is here,
I love him so much and will protect him so dear;
I am here for my dancers! I'll reply at no cost.
If only you knew how I feel guilty and lost!

I'm a teacher of dance, I feel exhausted and low,
I love time with my baby, but I need you to know,
I am here for my dancers, and I feel a strong pull,
I want you to know that my heart is so full!

I'm exhausted, I'm tired, I want it to stop!
I love to dance! I love to teach – so wait! I can't stop!
I am here for my dancers, and my heart is at home.
I don't know what to do, but I feel all alone!

I'm a teacher of dance and I've stopped feeling sad.
I love dance, I love home, no need to feel bad.
It's not my son's thing, but my daughter loves dance,
I still love to teach, and I still love to dance!

Head up, shoulders back, let's dance for our hearts!

## A message to my younger self...

If I could go back in time and speak to my younger self,
I would say that you are worth investing in and you are
stronger than you realise. You have so much to offer others,
and don't be afraid to tell people. You are hard-working,
clever, funny, kind, thoughtful, and passionate. You! Yes,
you!

You are also stubborn, sensitive, impatient, and feisty, when it involves any injustice. Embrace all of these qualities. This is you being you and there is no need to change!

You have so much to be grateful for, but it is sometimes necessary to ask for help, too! You really are going to be okay, but you have to share your worries and struggles to be able to move forward and find calm at the end of the chaos! It is absolutely fine to say goodbye to anything that is bringing any negativity your way.

You are important, you do matter, and people care!

You really need a hug, and I just want to squeeze you and tell you to believe in yourself! Please try not to take other people's comments to heart. They are mostly making assumptions, and they do not understand what is happening in your life and any struggles you may be working on. Their advice is often coming from a good place.

You are sensitive and try to hide your feelings, because you feel ashamed. It doesn't mean you're not feeling sad; it just stops you sharing your worries and emotions. This also causes you to be easily affected by people's words and actions. But please remember that when people mock or criticise, it is usually about what *they* may be going through. Make sure you talk to people.

I wish I had known that there is no need to feel guilty about self-care and no shame in asking for help. Both are so important for our mental and physical health.

Being able to survive everything I have been through has shown me that I am strong and determined, and that finding the people who will cheer us on and motivate us is so important. Life is too precious and too short to let other people's fears and beliefs stop us from moving forward and caring for ourselves. It is time to do what your heart is telling you to do! Be your authentic self!

I now feel able to listen to my heart. I feel proud for working on myself to be the best that I can be as a mum and as a businesswoman.

I am so grateful, so happy, and realising my self-worth more and more! When you realise your own self-worth, you can truly smile!

*I am The Girl Who Refused to Quit.*

## Dedication

To my beautiful babies, Finn and Orla, who keep me motivated and remind me to keep smiling and laughing.

To David, my amazing husband, you encourage, inspire and motivate me every day, more than you realise. I love you so much and love how much you make our little family smile!

To my parents who introduced me and encouraged me with my love of Irish dancing.

## About the Author

Natalie, who lives in Kent, England, is mostly described as a gentle, friendly and sensitive soul, who dislikes injustice and unkind behaviour!

When she's not helping people with their design needs, or with health and wellness through aloe vera products or

Irish dancing, she can be found relaxing with her family.

She is a very proud to be studying for her NLP (Neuro-Linguistic Programming) Master Practitioner Certification and EFT & TFT Tapping Practitioner Certification to be able to help her dancing students with their positive mindset and self-belief, which can be challenged when putting themselves out on a stage to be critiqued and judged!

Natalie's mission is to help others realise that it is OK to ask for help, no matter how big or small the problem seems.

## Contact

To find out more about Natalie's forthcoming book, 'Dance For Your Heart – Finding Freedom' you can contact her here …

Email: alwayskindandbeautiful@outlook.com

Health & Wellness Facebook Group: https://www.facebook.com/groups/alwayskindandbeautiful/

Instagram: natkd_alwayskindandbeautiful

Dancing Facebook Page: https://www.facebook.com/hackettkyne/

# Open Your Eyes
## Chrissy Adcock

The date is March 18th, 2020, and people are acting like the world is ending, due to a virus called Covid-19!

But guess what? My world had already ended five years ago! Or so I thought…

The 7th of March, 2015, was the day I realised that the world as I knew it would never be the same, when I heard the words, 'Are we there yet, Mom?' We pulled up to the forest where I had planned an adventure day out for just me and my boys, who were then five and six. As we walked up to the activity centre, I could hear children shouting and screaming. These were sounds of happiness and not the other kind. Oh my days, this is starting to sound like a scene from a horror story… but it's okay… we were at *Go Ape* forest adventure.

We signed in, and as we were waiting for our time slot, the boys went off and played in the play area. It was around midday, and I was surrounded by happy families. Everywhere I looked I could see moms prepping the perfect picnics while the dads laughed and joked about with their kids, throwing the little ones three feet up in the air and catching them. This made me feel sad, as I remembered back to when the boys' dad used to do this, and it would scare the shit of me.

It was at that precise moment when I realised that my and the boys' lives would never be the same again. I would never watch their dad do that to them again; I'd never feel that wave of fear or feel scared that he was going to drop them, because from now on I'd be the one doing it. I'd be the one doing everything – the fun, crazy, adventurous stuff, as well as the boring everyday mommy stuff. From now on, I would have to play both mom and dad roles. And no, their dad isn't dead or in the boot of my car, and I definitely hadn't planned to bury him in that same forest. Although, as a woman who'd had her trust betrayed for months, I might have visualised it once or twice! Oh, I'm going back to horror story mode – I've no idea where it's coming from; the words are just flowing!

So, let's go back a few months to October 2014. It was Hallowe'en – my favourite time of year, I may add! It's my birthday month, and back then I had a bright orange 1970's VW fastback car that we called 'Pumpkin' (I'll come back to that in a minute). I was an absolute mess, completely heartbroken, and sleeping alone in the spare room of our family home.

After two months of suspicion, due to disappearing acts, missed phone calls, secret messages, and even staying out all night, I knew he was seeing someone else. I had people telling me what was going on, but I refused to accept it. I didn't want to accept it; he was the love of my life and the father of my two wicked, awesome boys.

We had plenty of heated discussions about it, when he'd say he loved both of us, and that he didn't know what to do. I even chucked her out my house, followed by the heart-shaped chocolate cake that she made him for his birthday. How could someone rock up on the doorstep of a family home with a fucking heart-shaped cake for the man of the house? Knowing I'd answer the door and knowing the children were in the house? Knowing she was breaking up a family?

I couldn't eat. I couldn't sleep. I was in this zombie-like state where I had no idea what to do! It wasn't until one morning, when I'd come home from a night out in Birmingham with my bestie Jade, my son Oakley said to me, 'Mommy, Emma slept in your bed.' That was it! I moved out of the master bedroom and into the spare room. I had finally accepted that this was the end of our ten-year relationship.

So there I was, broken on the floor, leaning up against my single bed, surrounded by car parts and other random shit that ends up in a spare room, crying my eyes out, and feeling numb. I could hear the boys laughing and playing in their rooms. This would usually be the part of the story where ★POOF★ a fairy godmother appears. But, sorry to break it to you, life ain't no fairy-tale! There's no crazy magic lady to wave a stick to make everything hunky-dory again. It was down to me, and ONLY ME. I had to find my own power and be strong for my boys!

Suddenly I remembered it was going to be Hallowe'en soon and we always had fun and decorated the house. I thought, *Sod that, this ain't my home any more* (as he had already been moving her in), *so instead we are gonna decorate 'PUMPKIN'* (our orange 1970s car). I dried my eyes, went in the loft, and pulled down all the decorations before shouting happily, 'Come on, boys, let's go and decorate the car!'

We put cobwebs everywhere inside – apart from the windscreen, because I still needed to drive them to school. There was a Happy Hallowe'en banner on top of the windscreen, pumpkins on the back shelf, and glow-in-the-dark ghosts hanging off the indicator stems! We had sooo much fun doing it, and yes, I did drive them to school in it every single day for the whole of October.

And do you know what? They still remember that day. Even though they must have sensed what was going on, that will be a great memory forever, and when/if they ever do read this, I want them to know that even through my darkest days they were my strength. Who needs a fairy godmother when you have two amazing boys?

## Moving out!

You know that awful feeling when your chest tightens, a lump appears in the back of your throat, and it becomes really hard to talk without bursting into tears? Yeah, this is exactly how I felt as my ex-partner and I told the boys that our relationship had ended and that I was moving out. Watching six-year-old Oakley's bottom lip quiver and his eyes fill up with tears was devastating. It took every ounce of my energy to hold it together. I didn't want this to happen; I couldn't actually believe this was happening. I was literally dying inside just watching his reaction and answering his question, 'Will we see you, Mommy?'

You may be wondering why did I have to move out

of our family home? Guys, how was I supposed to live in the house that I had bought with the love of my life? All the memories that came with it and the pain of how it all ended, were just too much. I had to get away. I had to get out. And yes, of course, the boys came with me and would visit their dad on a regular basis. Luckily, a family member was able to help with the finances. Even though this whole situation broke her heart, she helped me to leave and I'm forever grateful for that.

So, I got the keys to our new house on the 6th December, 2014. A house which, may I add, 'he' (my ex) actually helped me find. Writing this now, I'm thinking, *What the actual fudge?! This whole situation was so screwed.* But I didn't know how to handle it or what to do. I was still in love with the guy! I was only 17 when we first met. I had no idea about what made a good house, and I had never made a decision on my own before; he had always been there.

One decision I did make was that the boys and I would move out on Christmas Day! I made sure the whole house was set up. I bought second-hand bunkbeds, and thankfully pretty much everything else, like a TV, sofa, and cupboards, were all given to me. Everything had to be ready so that the move was seamless.

I didn't want to spoil their Christmas, and as he had decided to go to his new girlfriend's parents' house for Christmas dinner, I decided that we would all spend Christmas morning together as a family, then the boys and I would go to Nanny and Grandad's for our meal and back to our new house.

This worked out really well. I knew I would be able

to hold myself together on Christmas Day so that it didn't spoil things for the boys. It was a whole new and different adventure and it helped that the boys absolutely loved their new room and the bunkbeds. It was an extra special Christmas present, and the start of our new life as a family of three.

## Let's go camping

As soon as spring came, I took the boys to get our own camping gear. We had always done the odd Volkswagen festival, and I knew the boys loved it. A lot of my friends were in the scene, so it made it easier for me to go and see people and to socialise.

Our first show with just the three of us was at a local small charity VW show. My mates, who ran a free VW magazine, had a stall there and they gave me a free ticket in return for helping them on the stall. Perfect! The boys could go off and play with their mates and have their own freedom. I'm not gonna lie – this scared the shit out of me, as I was relying on them to stay together and look out for one another, and to be back at a certain time. THEY HAD NO PHONES. But it was all good. Everything worked out.

Darwin only came back once on his own, because apparently the others had gone too far and out of bounds. I told him, 'To be honest, babe, I'd prefer you all stick together rather than wondering round on your own.' So, for the rest of the year – actually every year up until 2018 – every weekend, we went camping!

We were hardly ever in the house. It's only looking back and writing this that I'm thinking, *Wow! I have literally been running away and keeping busy!* It didn't help that I'd never really felt settled in that house, or anywhere else for that matter. I never put pictures up in that house or in our 'family home'.

When the boys did go to their dad's, I did everything I could to be out of the house. I hated being there alone. Even when they were at school, I'd go out of my mind. I just felt so lost. I'd also go to the shops and spend money faster than it was coming in, and on things we didn't necessarily need (mainly food). I'd never buy clothes or anything for me. I was just looking for something to do.

I had no job, but didn't really need one financially, as thankfully my rent was paid and I had benefits to live on. I was actually way better off than ever before. But there was still something missing.

I didn't know what to do with myself. I started looking at going back to college, but nothing seemed to fit. Everything I had started before, I had quit either because I couldn't seem to get my head around the subject or I was shit at writing and the theory side of things. (Who would have thought I'd be writing a sodding book? Ha ha!)

Eventually, I found a part-time cleaning job, which fit around school hours and I'd be earning more money. Or so I thought. Actually, it turned out I was worse off, and ended up being stuck in a job I hated. So I kept looking.

For some reason, I found myself scrolling through Facebook one day and came across a travel business opportunity to work from home. I didn't even like being at home, but I knew I wanted to travel more and that I hated my current job. So, I looked into it and, even though at the time I didn't have money to invest, I took the leap. The boys and I lived on beans on toast for a week as a result, but they loved it. It meant that I could start my business working from home and within the biggest industry on the planet. I love to travel, and I was sooo excited to get started! But little did I know what a whole new world it would open up! Oh, my days!

## Book Club

I had no idea what the hell network marketing was or that I had even signed up for it. All I knew was that I had my own travel business where I could earn money back on my travel and have the opportunity to earn money by sharing it with others. I went on a team Zoom call where my upline manager set us a book challenge. I explained that I didn't read, and that I found it really hard because I would have to read the same page about four times before it stuck in my head. She introduced me to Audible, and I humoured her and got my free 30-day trial with every intention of deleting the app after that time.

OH NO, that's not what happened. After listening to the first book, I was hooked. I then went on to listen to twelve more books that year. And all whilst working at that shitty cleaning job that I thought I hated. Now I'm extremely grateful for that job, because I wouldn't be the person I am today, writing this book, with the hope of inspiring you and showing that no matter what has happened in your life you CAN still achieve your dreams! You can still turn things around!

So yeah, I'm a massive believer that things happen for a reason, and it's only recently that I have taught myself the art of self-reflection and acknowledging (it took me ages to work out how to spell that, sitting sounding the letters out, ha ha!) my feelings. Whilst writing this, I've realised that I have just been in pure flight mode for the past five years! I've been doing everything I thought I wanted – keeping busy, taking every opportunity I could to keep moving forward but to never actually stop, reflect, and think. Although, if I hadn't done any of those things or met the people I met, I wouldn't be sitting here in the kitchen of my new family home, with my new fella, writing this book.

Everything really does work out as it should. And I've learned that this whole situation and what I thought was the end of the world was actually the beginning of a blessing in disguise.

It pushed me to find out who I really am – almost as if a rocket got shoved up my arse. Or going back to the fairy-tale analogies, maybe this sleeping beauty woke up from a long ass sleep and it took her so-called prince to give her a massive slap in the face instead of a kiss. Okay, that is not the way the fairy-tale goes, but when have I ever done things by the book? I'm writing my own darn book now, so this one maybe this is the exception as I literally re-write my future.

The point I'm trying to make is that everyday I'm slowly becoming more me. I'm not doing things the way other people expect me to; I'm doing things my way. I'm no longer living the 'ladder life', where you get the man, the house (which he chose), the car (which he chose), the children, the perfect job, and live happily ever after, and if you don't get these things you are always looking for them. Or even when you have these things, you still look for something more – the promotion, the newest car, the new skin lotion that has an irresistible almond scent.

I'm not a materialistic person at all, but some people are and that's fair enough. However, if you always looking for the next thing, you are never going to be happy. I've found that happiness is about what you're pursuing in the moment and the experiences you have. You've got to follow your heart and do what you wanna do, because happiness really does come from within.

Of course, I have the perfect experience of my own to back this up. Remember 'Pumpkin', my bright orange 1971 VW fastback? Well, I sold it… and immediately there was a massive shift in my energy, in confidence, and in my HAPPINESS! I'll tell you why. Getting my driving licence at the age of seventeen was the best thing I ever did, and being on the road and driving is my happiest place of all. But I noticed a pattern ever since I bought my first car. It was a 1997 lilac Renault Clio and I loved it, but I wanted the bright yellow classic Beetle that I was told I couldn't have, because it was too old and 'not ideal' as my first car.

Every car I ever owned up until June 2019 was one that had been chosen for me or given to me – even Pumpkin. I have always wanted to live on the road and go on adventures, but I kept a hold of Pumpkin for so long (seven years) because I was told it was part of my identity and that I couldn't get rid of it. So, when I sold him last year, even though I was sad to see him go, I was also extremely happy because I was buying something for me and only me – Rafiki, my VW T4 camper van! It felt like a massive 'Fuck you!' to everyone! A declaration that I'm doing things my way and I don't give a shit what anyone thinks. I'm happy, so you can shove your opinions where the sun don't shine!

So yeah, no more living in others' expectations; no more ladder life; I'm no longer looking for the next thing; I'm no longer lost. And all this is because of making one decision – well, actually loads of little decisions that have moved me forward, aka the compound effect.

These daily decisions have made me a stronger and better version of myself. The pivotal point was starting to read books, as this has expanded my knowledge and my self-awareness. So, if you too are struggling, you are off to a great start by reading this book right now! When you're done, make the decision to read some more, and I hope you will also discover that you don't need a fairy godmother to find your inner power and to change your life!

## Recommended Reading

*You Are a Badass* – Jen Sincero
*The 5 Second Rule* – Mel Robbins
*Girl, Wash Your Face* – Rachel Hollis
*Open Your Eyes* – Chrissy Adcock (Coming soon!)

## A message to my younger self...

If I could go back in time and speak to my younger self, I would want to tell her… Oh my days, YES, it is hard right now. Yes, everything hurts! Yes, you feel lost and alone, but everything is going work out as it's supposed to, I promise. Because I tell you now, you and only you have the power to change your life. So, get off your butt and take some action! Show your children the right way. Show them resilience, show them to fight back, show them that you are not giving up!

Girl, firstly, knowledge is power. Yes! Self-development is an actual thing and it's extremely important! I know you don't like to read, but get out your own ass, there are other ways. Listening to other people's stories and learning from their experiences is priceless. Learn about the Law of Attraction, expand your horizons, open your eyes! Don't be scared of what people think or the way they are doing things. When everything aligns with you and everything that you stand for, it doesn't matter what people think. Everything just flows and you are being you. So, if it doesn't feel right, then it's not. Just go with your gut! Figure out what energises you, work out what makes you happy in every moment, and follow that. You have got this!

I wish I had known that after everything you'll be much stronger than you ever thought you could be, and you will not be afraid to be you! Because it's okay to stand out. You don't have to follow the normal And you don't have to have a 'normal' family that all stays together. Children grow up in broken homes and they turn out just fine. (Well, I'm still clinging onto that one, as they are still only eleven and twelve!)

But, still speaking as your future self, after going through everything and still going through shit right now (sorry to say, it doesn't get easier; there's always a challenge), I feel as though I have the tools and the knowledge (if I don't have it, I can find it) to get through anything life throws at me. SO, LISTEN TO ME, DAMNIT! Right now, I feel empowered and freaking amazeballs, because I know that it's down to me to change things if I'm not happy. One decision is all it takes to swing me in the right direction, which ultimately makes me in control of my own life and my own mind! (Well, most of the time anyway; lady hormones do take over every month, but hey, I am a woman!)

I am a strong, confident, unstoppable woman. I am ME!

*I am The Girl Who Refused to Quit.*

## Dedication

To Oakley and Darwin you both are my strength, my strength to get through the tough times and to keep on going no matter what!

And to Chris Watkins you have given me the extra push, the courage and the support I needed to share my story!

## About the author

Chrissy Adcock lives in Worcestershire England. She has been described as kind empathetic supportive soul with the guts and will to succeed at whatever her heart desires

When she's not booking travel and inspiring others to

be the best version of themselves, she can be found on the road in her van having crazy ace adventures.

She is a very proud momma of two boys (mentioned above) who keep her on her toes and give her the strength to keep striving for better every day.

Her mission is to show them and everyone that they have to power to achieve their dreams! To show them that anything is possible!

## Contact

Facebook: @chrissyadcock86
Chrissyadcock86@gmail.com
https://www.youtube.com/channel/UC4hX_Mcoa2LA5
  ef6mNLYiWg

# The Pink Slippers

*Sally Dawson*

## *So it begins…*

'No! I'm not F…ing going!' I shouted. 'Everyone will know.'

'They won't,' my sister gently replied.

'Look at me, how will they not know? I'm not normal any more!' I was standing in my kitchen with tears streaming down my face as my partner came over to me, put his arms lovingly around me, and encouraged me to go with my sister. Knowing he had an important meeting that he had to be at in the next thirty minutes, he didn't shout, he just stayed calm, and spent the next fifteen minutes, along with my sister, gently convincing me to get into the car.

Eventually, I agreed on one condition. If I was leaving the house, then I would be going in my bright pink slippers! 'No problem,' my sister replied with a look that can only be described as a mixture between a grin and a grimace!

So, with plenty of cajoling and me defiantly dressed in my jeans, jumper, and bright pink slippers, I finally got into the car. Our journey wasn't long – only ten or fifteen minutes – but despite my sister not knowing where to go, I just sat in the car staring out of the window, thinking and reflecting about the last few months and how had I got to this point.

All too soon, we arrived at the hospital. Tears filled my eyes again as I got out of the car and walked – well, to be fair, shuffled – towards the building in my pink slippers. We made our way down the corridor and my sister stopped to check me in at the reception.

'Take a seat,' the receptionist said, with a smile and a sympathetic look in my direction. As time goes on you do eventually get used to the looks and the cock of the head, but not today. This was by far my biggest fear – everyone knowing, looking at me, and just knowing that I was different.

Tears continued to run down my face as the silent sobs threatened to come again. 'F– this, I'm not doing this.' I stood up to go home, but my sister just gently tugged me to sit down.

We sat there in silence. To be honest, my sister was probably talking, but I wasn't really listening. My name was called and one of the most amazing people I was going to meet on this journey then came over, lent down, and gently touched my arm.

'Ready?' she asked.

'Not really…' I replied, as my tears continued to fall.

'Let's have a look and see how we are doing,' she said.

I followed her down another corridor to a small room, and took a deep breath. This was it. My sister offered to wait outside, but I needed her now more than ever, so asked her to come in. Once again, panic set in. *What would*

*my sister think of me? Would she think I was the freak I felt?*
Looking back now, the reason everyone was staring at me
as I walked down those corridors was because of my choice
of footwear, nothing else!

Nurse Mandy asked me to take my top off, including
my bra. She helped me to undress, and moved the medical
draining bag that I was carrying around with me. As I sat on
the hospital bed, she looked down at my feet and, smiling,
said, 'Nice slippers.'

I smiled back as my sister explained the reason for
them.

'Whatever makes you comfortable,' she replied. 'This is
your journey, no-one else's.'

I took a deep breath and looked down at the
uncomfortable tubes and stitches. You see, instead of a
perfectly, or even imperfectly-shaped boob, I now had a
cut – a great big ugly mark where my boob should have
been.

As the breast care nurse checked everything over, she
explained that my scar was healing well but they couldn't
remove the drain as I still had too much fluid. She asked
how I was finding the pain factor and if I was coping okay
with the soft prosthesis. All these matter of fact questions
continued, and the whole time I was looking down at those
bloody pink slippers.

Suddenly I had the realisation that I was wearing pink
for breast cancer, and it was all just too much. I broke down
again for what seemed like the 100th time that day, and just
sobbed and sobbed.

You may think that my confidence meltdown would
have come when I was told at the age of 40 that I had breast

cancer. But no, my meltdown came three months later – four days after I lost my right breast.

My journey started in 2012 when I noticed a small lump on my right boob. Nothing major, I didn't worry, it was just there. It was my partner who convinced me to go to the doctor. The doctor didn't appear concerned, but to be on the safe side decided to refer me to the hospital. I went along one Thursday morning, not thinking or worrying about it; I even took my mom with me for company, arranging to go for lunch afterwards. How very optimistic of me!

For anyone who has never been to a Breast Care Clinic, the experience is rather unique. Firstly, you go with the nurse, get weighed, height checked, and it's all jovial. Then you go through and wait for your consultant, meet the breast care nurses, who turn out to be the most amazing people you will ever meet. Then you meet your consultant. I'm not a prude in any way, shape, or form, but yes, initially it's a little embarrassing getting your boobs out for various different strangers. I can honestly say by the end of my journey, so many people had seen my boobs that I wasn't – and am still now – not that bothered. I would happily walk down the street topless if it meant this disease no longer existed!

So, off I went to meet the consultant. He was lovely and felt all around and gave me a large brown envelope then sent me to the X-ray department for a mammogram. After a little while, they sent me to have an ultrasound and then for a chest X-ray. By this time you have been there for about three hours, had a couple of cups of crappy coffee, and then you go back to see the consultant, who sits you down with the breast care nurses – and your large brown envelope is on the desk.

Over the many weeks of sitting in the breast clinic, Thursday after Thursday, you begin to empathise with anyone with a brown envelope walking towards the X-ray department. You wonder if you will see them the next week, or maybe they will get lucky and the big brown envelope is just a red herring on this occasion. It's amazing what goes through your mind as you sit there, waiting, smiling, pretending…

I digress – something I do quite often. I suspect it's a coping mechanism; see I'm off again! The next conversation I had is still a blur in my mind. It was as though I was stuck in a bad dream as I was told there were definitely nodules and they had concerns about certain areas. I was handed leaflets about breast cancer, lumpectomies and mastectomies, and informed that I would need a biopsy.

I just sat there, not really taking it in. They asked if I understood and I nodded like a numb robot, not really understanding anything they had said. The breast care nurse took me into a side room with my mom so I could catch my breath, and asked if I needed to call anyone. I got my phone out to call my partner, Kevin, but when he answered I fell apart.

My mom, as moms do, just took control of the situation. She explained to Kev what they had said, got me in the car, and somehow got me home in one piece. Needless to say, we never got to have our lunch that day! I walked into the house and into the arms of one of the most amazing people I'm lucky enough to have in my life. Kev held me close whilst I sobbed, trying to get my words out as I explained what the hospital had said.

When you're told they think you have cancer, you feel

numb, you don't really take it all in. And then you're given a glimmer of hope – only a small one, but still a tiny ray of light. You get a call or a letter to arrange the next step, so off you go to the hospital to have a biopsy. This is to confirm how bad, how advanced this God-awful disease is in you, yet still somewhere you think they may have got it wrong, they might just have made a mistake. After all, this is to confirm everything, isn't it?

The biopsy itself is another rather strange experience. You go to have an X-ray and then you start with another ultrasound. Now, I've never had a baby of my own, but I would imagine it is both joyful and a little bit frightening waiting to hear your baby's heartbeat. Well, this is a bit like waiting for a bright pink neon light to start flashing 'cancer', or singers and dancers to come in singing your own little song, 'She has cancer, she has cancer', and then everyone starts applauding, didn't she do well!

Okay, so that never happens, but if you're fortunate you get a lovely doctor who sees how distressed you are and allows your partner to be with you. They then go on to explain that this f...ing great big needle is going to be inserted into your boob, but it's okay as they are going to numb the area first with a much smaller needle. If you're okay with needles, that's fine, but I'm really not. Kev's fingers were pretty squished at this point.

And then comes the noise. As they click to take the sample, it sounds like a really loud stapler, and they ask you to be completely still and try not to move. Yeah, that's really easy to accomplish, not!

So, after they have taken four samples, you get to go home and wait for the results, which has to be the most tense time you will experience. With the exception of my mom and dad, my best friend, and my sisters, no-one was aware of what was going on. Your emotions are through the roof – one minute you're angry, the next you are in tears. I wouldn't tell work or my friends; if I didn't say it out loud then it couldn't be happening.

Unfortunately, they too were struggling with my impending results, and I ended up having about four separate biopsies. At one stage I had titanium put in my boob so they could see where they had taken the samples from. I was covered in bruises, and when I was sent for another mammogram, the pain was unbelievable as they squeezed my boob into the machine and blood was pouring out of the wounds.

I sort of floated through the next couple of weeks. Kev as ever was by my side every step of the way, and between him, my dogs, and my best friend, we made it to results day. Kev had already asked me what my worst fear was, and I realised that it was to be told that I was riddled with it and they couldn't save me. I was forty and happy; I had found love again; I had survived a bad marriage; I had survived insurmountable debt; I had survived the divorce from hell. And now, when I was finally settled and happy and loved unconditionally, I was petrified that I was going to die from an f…ing lump in my boob!

As the appointment got ever nearer, my fear and anxiety just went through the roof. I even went to work in the morning, thinking it would help my focus. Spoiler alert, it was a really bad idea. Colleagues, not knowing or understanding, didn't come within ten metres of my desk for fear of being politely asked to bugger off!

Eventually the time arrived to start my journey of doom. I met Kev at home, cuddled my dogs, and off we went. I arrived, gave my name, and watched people disappear with that dreaded brown envelope. It all felt surreal, a bit like an out-of-body experience; I sort of floated everywhere. They called my name and again the breast care nurses were there, waiting to hold my hand and offer comfort.

My consultant started talking and my world stopped spinning. I heard snippets of words like, 'I'm sorry to tell you… it has been confirmed… you have stage…' and then the big word, the capital letter you never want to hear, 'Cancer'.

I looked round for that neon sign or the dancing girls and singers, but they weren't there. Just me, Kev, the consultant, and the nurse.

'Did you read the leaflets I gave you?' I heard this voice asking. 'Yes.' I guess it was me answering. I didn't really hear anything past that, I think I just nodded, we left, set another appointment for the following week for a treatment plan, and walked out of the hospital.

Kev just looked at me and asked if I wanted to take a minute, but I shook my head. I just wanted to go home to my dogs. I fumbled in my bag for the car park ticket, and the machine flashed up at me that we owed £2.50. I chose that moment to let loose. '£2.50!' I shouted. '£2.50 to be told I've got f…ing cancer! £2.50, are you kidding me?' For those that know the garlic bread scene of a well-known comedian, you can now imagine me in a car park, shouting £2.50 over and over at the top of my voice, and people just taking a wide berth as they walked past.

We drove home in a daze. Kev asked me if I understood

what they had said, and I realised I hadn't taken any of it in. After that, Kev recorded all our appointments on his phone so that I could listen back afterwards and digest all the information. I don't think you are officially allowed to do this, but it really helped me and, un-beknown to me, Kev would listen and research things after I had gone to bed so that he understood everything and could try to answer my many questions.

We then had the horrific task of telling people the news. I couldn't face my mom and dad, as I somehow felt I had failed them, so I started with my best friend. It's both a comfort and extremely painful listening to your best mate fall apart on the phone, but she was, as always, amazing. I heard the sharp intake of breath and then she rose again and said all the right things, about how we were going to beat this and how we were going to get through.

After finding the words to tell the family, next came my stepdaughter, Rebecca. I'm lucky to be extremely close to her, so I get the best of both worlds of being a mom and a friend. We decided it was best for Kev to tell her on his own. I think it was so that he didn't have to deal with the two of us crying! Kev went to collect her from her mom's and gently explained what had happened, and I think it was the only time he let a few tears out. The rest of the time, he held everything together for me. Rebecca came running in the house and just cuddled me. She doesn't really do cuddles, so this was the real deal, and incidentally, it was Rebecca who bought me the memorable pink slippers.

I can't write this book without mentioning my two dogs. Our Rottweiler and Basset Hound both became my crying pillows when I was on my own; the Basset used to lie on my tummy and I would just stroke his ears, and the Rottweiler was always by my side. Kev would often come home and find me asleep with my head on the Rottweiler, and the Basset Hound asleep on my stomach! Sadly, I have now lost both of them. But at the time, along with my slippers, they were my comfort blankets.

After the emotional rollercoaster of those couple of weeks, I thought things would be more structured. So, when we went to my next appointment, I had a clear plan. Unfortunately, though, this was my plan not the consultant's!

He asked if I understood what the next step would be, and I quite loudly and clearly announced that I would have a lumpectomy please. I thought it was a bit like choosing from a menu, looking at your options, and deciding what took my fancy!

My consultant calmly explained that I would need a mastectomy. I replied, politely and clearly, that I would like a lumpectomy please.

'Miss Dawson,' he said, 'this is not open for negotiation. You have to have a mastectomy.'

No way! 'I'm forty, and I don't want one,' was my response. 'I'm not going to have a body without a boob. Why can't I have a lumpectomy? I choose a lumpectomy; it's there on the menu choices, that's what I want.' I could hear my voice getting louder, my anger and my tears mixing into one as Kev's hand gently stroked mine, trying to get me to be calm.

Then came the double blow. 'We're not clear if it's isolated,' the consultant said. 'Your tumour is at least 6cm long and we need to ensure we get everything.

Unfortunately, you will also need a small operation to remove and test your lymph nodes, as we think it may have spread. There was also some concern of a lump in the other breast.'

What! Why had this gone so wrong? My simple plan of a lumpectomy had gone out the window, and so it began with the tests, the operation, my journey of hell, my refusal to accept what I was being told, and my unwanted tour of every breast care unit in the West Midlands.

So, this is just the beginning of my story, as my true journey began with a pair of bright pink slippers and it won't end until I get to throw them away…

# A message to my younger self…

If I could go back in time and speak to my younger self, I would want to give her some simple advice. Firstly, always trust in yourself; your gut reaction and your instincts are your greatest tools. Learn to use them and trust your initial feelings.

We don't believe in regrets; we never have and never will. The pain and the upset that you will feel is something you need to go through in order to come out the other side.

Take a deep breath and slowly release, accept the good, the bad and the ugly, as they all go hand-in-hand. You will get through this. Your strength, your stubbornness, your damn right pig-headedness will show you the way, and when you emerge from this trauma and this journey, you will have learned from it.

Let the tears fall; you will need to cleanse your body and your mind of negativity. Along with the tears will come the anger. Let it loose. Remember, as with the tears, it needs to be released, so shout at the top of your voice whenever you want, don't care what people think, don't care that people may look. Let them look, let them stare, this is your journey to travel not theirs! Don't hold the negativity in, trust and release. And don't push away those that love you. Accept the love and help offered by those around you; there are times when they will become your voice.

Stand your ground when you need to and fight for what you believe is right for you. Ultimately, you might not get what you want, but you will learn from it and you need to learn to find your path within the healing world.

For every cloud has a silver lining... This will become your mantra; remember it and shout it out loud when you need to feel better about yourself. This path will also lead you to Reiki. You will learn how to use Reiki for your own self-healing, and you will learn now to offer this wonderful therapy to other people. The principles of Reiki will eventually become your new mantra, so don't fight this wonderful tool you will be offered. Embrace it, learn from it, and move forward with it.

Love those slippers. They will become your comfort zone, along with your scarf, and you will use them to hide behind, cry into, and to help you through the darkest of days.

And most importantly, love yourself. Sometimes you need to go through your fear to see the beauty on the other side.

So, girl, when the time comes to throw out those pink

slippers, drink champagne and dance on the table. Go for it!

I am lucky. I am blessed. I am a survivor.

*I am The Girl Who Refused to Quit.*

## Dedication

To Kevin, my love, my light, my soul you held my hand through the toughest of times, caught my tears on the hardest days. Together we stood, side by side, hand in hand, shoulder to shoulder and battled the good, the bad and the ugly times. We came out the other side still smiling and holding hands. All my love x

## About the author

Sally lives in Redditch, Worcestershire, she is a Reiki Master, a Reflexologist and is currently working towards her qualifications in many other holistic therapies. She is often described as a hard working, dedicated and a loving individual who will do anything to help others, her cup is always half full and brimming over. When not working Sally can often be found walking with her partner and two dogs or enjoying her caravan in Evesham. She loves to read Oracle Cards especially Angel, Animal and Unicorn cards.

Sally's offers holistic and colour healing and is working towards offering all her holistic gifts and training to individuals and families battling and recovering from

Cancer, her ultimate goal is to offer these treatments free of charge so patients can have some downtime and relaxation to help them through their ordeal and know they are never alone on their journey.

## Contact

Email. Sallyd71@hotmail.co.uk
Facebook / sally.dawson.794
Instagram sally.dawson.794

# Guided by the Light

## Elly Charles

*What the fuck just happened?* I slowly picked myself up from where I'd been lying on the pavement, as a stream of blood trickled out of my nose. In a daze, I slowly walked towards my friend Matt's house, where he stood in the doorway shaking his head with disbelief. My head pounded as I tried to work out how my night had started by having a few drinks in my local pub and ended by having the shit kicked out of me by a random woman I'd never met.

Why did she hate me so much? You guessed it; a man was involved. My ex-boyfriend, to be precise. We had split up a few months earlier but, rightly or wrongly, we had carried on sleeping together. I had no idea that he was seeing another woman, but she had found out and she wanted revenge. After many dirty looks and angry words in the pub, she found out where I lived and came to find me with two of her friends.

I had stopped at Matt's flat on my way home, but somehow, she still knew where I was. After hearing a loud knock, I opened the door and before I knew what was happening, I was being dragged into the street while Matt was held back by her friends. Initially, I had fought back, before asking myself, *Do I really want to fight over this man?* He had cheated on me, treated me like shit, and had not shown one inch of compassion when I'd had to make one of the hardest decisions of my life just a few weeks earlier.

They had gone now, but the memories hadn't. Matt cleaned up my face as I tried to make sense of it all…

Our relationship started at a time when my life was one big wild party. It was a raw, erratic relationship, with a lot of cheating and a lot of arguing, constant back and forth, treating each other like shit, pushing each other around while usually stupidly intoxicated. Pain, hatred, jealousy, out of control, the stuck feeling constantly whirled around in my head, on top of not realising that my drug taking was starting to get a hold of me. I was waking up each day, starting to lose myself more and more.

Darkness was all I saw. The darkness was deafening. The darkness was lonely. The darkness of drugs finds you in a very wrong world. The feeling of addiction is rife. Man, the mere thought of that feel-good vibe that the perfect powder brought me, yet the good vibe always wore off, if it came at all. The constant thoughts of cocaine turned into not wanting but needing this substance. I had gone from sniffing cocaine every few weeks to sniffing it every weekend and during the week.

I was stuck in this dark hole of sadness when I found out I was pregnant. How could I bring a baby into this world when I couldn't even look after myself? My (now ex) partner didn't seem to want this baby, and we weren't even together by this point. I saw myself as a fucked-up cokehead, so I made the decision to terminate my baby. Waiting an extra three weeks after booking the termination was excruciating. Knowing this little being was inside me, I felt so much love but so much pain. My baby deserved better then what I was; that's how I felt.

The night before my abortion, I stayed at my mum's house. I decided to speak to my baby. I knew she was a girl, because I could feel her energy, I could feel her listening. I told her, 'Little girl, I'm sorry that Mummy can't have you right now. You have to go back. I know you understand, little darling.' All I felt was immense love. She knew this was her path; she had come down to teach me a lesson.

I have cried writing this, because out of all the pain I have experienced, this was one of the hardest decisions of my life. Coming home after my termination, lying there knowing that her being was no longer in my belly, hurt like fuck. I was empty. She was gone.

My little girl in spirit regularly visits me to this day; she is mine forever. Thank you, my girl, for teaching me the lesson I needed. I will always love you. I see your beauty. I see your light…

'Ouch!' The lingering pain from being punched in the face brought me back to reality. It was almost unbearable, but it was nothing compared to the emotional pain in my heart. I was so grateful for Matt's help that night. He could see through the self-destruct mode I had ignited, and he always believed I would be okay. I wanted to believe in me, too, but could I really piece my life back together again when I had lost so much in such a short space of time?

After the attack, I became very scared and remained in my flat for months. I slept with a wooden bat next to the bed, and would often experience anxiety and bad nightmares. I realise now that this was mental health, yet back then there wasn't as much awareness about it. I was constantly looking over my shoulder, worrying that someone would come into my flat to hurt me. My bruised eyes and broken nose took time to heal, of course, but the emotional damage took a lot longer.

Gradually, I started to venture out again, but something had changed in me. I no longer wanted to argue with people, I no longer wanted drama. The transition of changing from full-on self-destruct mode into realisation mode was hard as hell, because now I started to understand all the shit that I had caused with my actions. I wanted to move forward with my life, but the noise in my head was dragging me down.

## *The Voices…*

Who are they? They scare me, these voices with different accents. Some sound like old people, some sound like children. Am I just hearing them because I'm on a comedown? They are all around me. The voices are closing in on me; my ears are buzzing and ringing from them.

Fuck the voices! They make me tired; they tell me stuff that I don't want to know. How do I know so much shit about random people I've just met? Because the voices tell me. Am I dead? Is that why I can hear them? Did I die and not realise? Oh my gosh, am I stuck in limbo?

Now, by this point in my life, it was no shock to me having spirits visit me daily. By then, I was very aware that I could speak to spirits. I had first discovered this when I was only four years old, but it wasn't until now, aged twenty-five, that I could hear, see and understand them. I could feel their pain from when they were alive. I fully understood the difference between dark spirit and light spirit. yet I was not at a stage of being able to clear spirit to the light.

I hadn't slept properly for a good year and felt like a walking zombie. I would struggle to sleep because of the voices and their presence within my bedroom and my personal space. 'Go away,' I would tell them, but they wouldn't leave. They'd rattle-rattle through my earrings hanging on the earring tree.

The feeling of being watched was powerful and I constantly battled with the realisation that through my drug-taking a few years back I had gained a whole lot of stuck spirits attaching to my energy. Back then, I hadn't realised it, because the feeling of the drugs overpowered the symptoms of these spirits hanging around me. Now years later, no longer taking drugs, these symptoms of spirit attachments were strong within me.

Some nights I would get ripped out of my bed by a presence so strong it was very scary; even hiding under the duvet or turning the light on wouldn't save me. Fear felt everlasting, and I used to hear this entity laughing and breathing in my ear. Eventually, my mum got me the training I needed, and a huge clearing was performed on me to release these dark spirits that haunted me so much. It's surprising how much these attachments trick you to believe that this is actually normal. I felt so much better after these entities were released.

After that, my Mediumship trainer and my mother taught me strong protection and grounding techniques, and I learnt how to control and filter every psychic message I was receiving. At that point I still in no way wanted to be a medium; I was afraid that I would pick up awful attachments or psychic attack. No, no, no. I was a photographer and that's what I wanted to continue doing. My trainers kept saying, 'Elly, in years to come you WILL be a medium and you WILL be helping people.' But I ignored those comments and resisted the pulls to learn psychically. I had no clue what was in store for me within the next few years.

I find it funny looking back now that for someone who is so very psychic, I was totally blind to see or believe in my future. I understand now of course, that if I had listened then I might not have tried or learnt the lessons I had to learn that became apart of my enlightenment. Sometimes our angels don't disclose the whole story to us. I get that now.

Enlightenment – oh, that word, I just love it. It's my favourite thing; the energy of enlightenment when it comes knocking can be so amazingly astounding. I love watching my students become more and more enlightened. You see, enlightenment is brought to you upon the transition path to your purpose path. Enlightened energy knows you will resist it, it knows you will question it, and it knows you will feel uncomfortable, but it also knows of THE RIGHT TIME, too. Enlightenment comes with the path that is bringing you alignment.

My transition continued and grew stronger when I finally decided to move to a completely different town. I had cut myself off from most of the friends I had shared drugs with, yet I was still addicted. I found myself in a lovely little flat, living on my own in a quiet area, and this is where my amazing healing and transformation began.

Over the coming months I found myself behaving in strange ways. I was absolutely skint, I had no job, no money, didn't have a clue how I would pay for my new home, and I was trying my hardest to keep myself locked indoors away from drugs or people I viewed as a bad influence.

I would find myself taking long baths and crying for hours. I would wash myself over and over, my warm tears dropping into the water. I'll never forget the smell of the bubble bath, which made me feel a little better. I also found that I would listen to music for hours. I would cry so much to Tracy Chapman's song *Fast Car*, because the words resonated with me.

## *Will this ever end?*

I would lie in the middle of the floor in my lounge and hug myself, then cry more. Sometimes I would feel angry and punch the wall or the floor, because I wanted to hurt my fist. It felt good.

I would get my mirror, place it against the wall, and sit and talk to myself. I would talk about everything that I had done, everything that had happened, and I would watch my face become red, my eyes welling up. Looking at the knife, I would roll the blade over my wrists and thighs, literally shaking my head so much that it was throbbing. I just couldn't do it; I couldn't kill myself. The mirror talking became a regular occurrence, yet over time, instead of telling myself 'I hate you', I started to say, 'Elly, I love you'. I started to look at myself in the mirror and say things

I liked about myself. Each time I was able to find more and more things that I liked about me.

Writing was another thing I found myself doing. I found it helped me when I wrote about my addiction. Gradually, over time I became clean from drugs, having gone four months with not one single sniff. I still thought about it every day, though, and battled that powder calling upon me.

In my sober days, this is when I really began to start talking to my angels. A few years before, my mum's best friend Mellie had passed away. And in this time of transformation and staying clean, I would sit in bed and speak out loud to Mellie, begging her to help me. I spoke to her because it felt more real to pray to her than to pray to God. I didn't know if she was listening, but it felt good to do it.

I cried so much to Mellie one night that I fell into a deep sleep. Waking up, I became aware of a beautiful glowing figure sitting on my bed looking at me. *Is that Mellie? Noooo, wait a minute, am I high? No, Elly, you have been clean for four months.* I just lay there still. *Oh, she's really there, El, she's fucking there.* The immense love I felt was so powerful.

She said, 'Why are you shocked, Elly? You asked for my help, it was only a matter of time before I came to you. It's time now, Elly. They have a plan for you. Follow my lead.' I asked Mellie what the plan was and who 'they' were, but she had gone. Yet I was left with the strong belief that I would somehow know what to do.

Mellie, you are so beautiful. You are my shining light. You have my back and I love you. My angel.

So, from when I was aged twenty-six to thirty, I found

the ways of healing, enlightenment, and trust. Mellie surely was right; she led me into alignment, taught me how to connect properly to spirit and to my guides, and taught me spiritual lessons. During this period, I had my daughter Minnie, met an amazing man who is her father, and I became more and more aware of what my destiny was and what their plan for me was. Fuck me, it was hard, but good. It's still unfolding. and I'm going with the flow.

I set up my spiritual business, Light After Life, and for the first time in my life I didn't have doubts. I began to understand more and more why I'd had so many years of pain and such a huge healing process, because actually I was meant to help others through my skillset. Suddenly, through my mediumship, I had more and more people booking to see me, and positive words being spoken about me. People wanted to hug me because I had brought them so much joy and comfort. People returned again and again, and over time I became so busy with my mediumship. It was fabulous and felt right, and any time I had a strong pull to try a new spiritual idea within my business, it would work with ease. I still didn't have any clue just how amazing this really was. People were publicly and positively recommending me, and I began to do readings for people across the country and all over the world. I began to realise this was the plan.

In this time, my lovely Grandmother Meryl passed away, and she has been the guiding force behind my business for the last two years. She kept visiting me, and told me to set up a class teaching spiritual development, which I – in typical human fashion – resisted for a while. I said, 'Grandma, I don't know how to set up a class, and I certainly don't know how to teach.'

Eventually Grandma pestered me so much that I finally gave in and set up a class. I thought I'd just see how it went. Fast forward two years to Elly, aged thirty-two, and that one class has now grown to eight different classes in various locations, including an online course, regular workshops, and teaching individual students.

The last two years have flown by. My partner worked long shifts late into the night, so I have managed to run my business to this level whilst doing all the motherly and household duties, too. You might ask how I did it and still continued to grow. Where has all this motivation come from? I used to be someone who didn't want to work, but now I'm someone who can't wait to wake up and work.

Well, my friends, it starts with a spiritual seed that was planted long before I was born and was written into my contract. We all walk our different lives, and we each have a different seed. The darkness and depression were all a part of my seed. When I started to heal, the healing energy watered that seed, which made me grow. Grow to understand the ever-expanding knowledge of the Universe. Grow to trust in my intuition and to know we are not alone.

Spirit is always supporting us. You see, I now know life is about ever-evolving. Life is for living.

It may have taken a long and painful journey to get here, but I now know that I am somebody who can get through anything. I am somebody who is brave; I am somebody that will continue to learn; I am somebody that can heal myself; I am somebody that trusts in the guidance from the Universe; I am a being of light; I am a Lightworker.

I let the light shine through me and guide me; the light protects me. I am somebody that helps people through my business. I am somebody that helps others by sharing my story.

## So, who am I?

I am Elly, and I am a transformer. I am Elly, and I now trust. I am Elly, and I am ever grateful for my journey of where I came from, what I've been through, and where I've got to. I am Elly, and Elly is energy, Elly is important, Elly is beautiful, Elly is a survivor and a thriver.

Elly is love.

Elly is me.

## A message to my younger self...

If I could go back in time and speak to my younger self, I would want to tell her...

Elly, you lovely little soul, shining so bright, so oblivious to what is about to happen. I now know that I would not change anything. That seems silly to say, because of the painful things that took place, but it's because I truly know that what has happened has brought me to my older self, where I am so understanding of just WHY I was treated so badly. I now know that this is my life, my story, and I can't change it, but I CAN forgive it.

I now understand that the pain I went through dimmed my shining light and blocked me in life. I was so lost for so long, my little heart felt like it wanted to stop beating and just give up on my life; the young side of myself became stuck within the energy of the older side of myself, which then presented so many fears and worries that made me feel so helpless in my older self.

I realised that YOU, ELLY, are my inner child and you needed healing. Thank you for being so strong when you were so young. Thank you for being so willing to overcome the darkness of the things you went through.

If I could go back, I would give her a huge sunflower to bring her happiness during the times that were so dark when she was six years old. I would put my arms around her and protect her from the man that did so many awful things to her body. I would remove any energy of his wrong-doings over her very being. I would tell her what she could do to protect herself, although I know why he was so horrid and now how she would become so strong within her mind and your body.

Elly, I am so proud of you and far you have come. I see your strength and your beauty, I see how you can forgive those that have hurt you. I hear you now.

I know that you are making miracles, I watched you ignite your light and start to come alive. I saw you bring back that light that shone so bright. Thank you for taking on your mission in life so young, even though you maybe did not realise back then what your mission was.

You see, in my dreams I saw the book of contracts shining so golden, given to me by a beautiful angel, and I knew that you had completed parts of your contract, I see that contract still now just further along the pages that were written for me, and I know there is still more to come. Now I know that by going through what I did enabled me to be able to conquer whatever is coming next within this beautiful contract.

Elly, you turned your pain into POSITIVE POWER.

I call this contract beautiful even if it's been full of pain and sorrow, because life is beautiful and, Elly, that's what you have taught me.

You taught me about remembering the small things in life through your darkest hours, things like the smell of freshly-cut grass made you feel better when you were all alone, or the thought that there is a light shining even if you couldn't see it any more. You also taught me to forgive myself. It was fucking hard, but you did it.

Thank you, Elly, for your truth.

Thank you, Elly, for the love so strong within your heart.

Thank you that your heart still beats.

Thank you for being alive.

You do matter, Elly.

Thank you for being you.

Thank you for igniting your light again.

Thank you for shining.

Thank you, thank you, thank you.

I am shining my light powerfully. I am trusting in the Universe.

I am The Girl Who Refused to Quit.


## Dedication

To my darling daughter Minnie Taylor, the day you arrived in my life was the day my life changed forever. You are the reason I keep going. You shine so bright and you are the love of my love. Thank you for being my daughter.

## About the author

Elly Charles is a positive, friendly young woman who just happens to be a psychic medium. She has a reputation for accuracy and has developed a wide psychic skill set, which means her readings are often profound and compassionate.

As well as being a busy mother, Elly also runs through her business Light After Life, psychic and spiritual development courses, workshops and retreats, as well as coaching. She feels her soul purpose is to support people to open up to a higher level of love bringing comfort, significance and clarity to the people she works with.

Elly comes from a family who for generations have had psychic and mediumship skills, using them for the good of all, so it is only natural that she began developing early. She learned from her mother and grandmother, who has since become one of her guides in spirit.

Elly believes that even through our darkest times, we are guided, we all just need a little support to light up the way sometimes.

## Contact

Facebook: /ellycharlesmediumship
Website: https://ellycharlesmediumship.com/
The School of Spirituality: https://ellycharlesmediumship.com/spirituality-2/
Instagram: https://www.instagram.com/lightafterlife

# Found in Transition

## Raychel Grace Paterson

*September 2017*

'No! I'm not gay… I'm bloody transgender!'

I was sitting at the kitchen table, shaking with the realisation of what I'd just admitted to, and yes, I felt an internal excitement that I'd done it. It was finally out in the open. But could I move on now, at last?

No sooner had the words left my mouth than I felt a crushing sense of impending doom. I wanted to take it back; it wasn't the right time to tell her. I'd needed to be in control of how and when, but she'd even robbed me of that pleasure. Stupidly, I questioned myself. *Can I not do anything right?* I felt like a child. *What was wrong with me?*

My partner's impenetrable expression told me everything I needed to know. Now I knew, without yet comprehending how, that my life would never be the same again. This was going to be both the hardest and yet the easiest challenge I was ever going to face. This was my truth. I felt that I'd been cheated of my birth right. A woman's body to match how I felt about myself deep inside. I have always known that despite being born as a man, I AM a woman.

On the rare times we had spoken in our relationship, it was only so that I could receive my daily instructions: Do this for me; do that for me. I felt like a slave. There was never any time for me to do me. None at all. I felt that she was watching me all the time, even when she wasn't there. She had to be MY top priority. The fact that I had always been a loner and lacking in social skills set the scene for a co-dependent relationship that was always going to be difficult, and became slowly toxic over time.

Barely ten minutes before the fateful, 'Are you gay?' question, I had been preparing for my night shift as a security guard. So, my head was all over the place when I was picked up by a colleague and taken to the site that evening. Saying nothing, I hid away in the duties of work that night, which wasn't hard. Mundane patrolling of a site that took little effort to look after. Anyone with half a brain could have done it. Hence, why I got the job. Ugh. I had to stop putting myself down.

For a whole week, nobody in the 'family' did or said anything. It was as if the conversation had never happened. People are strange, aren't they? Putting things off; sweeping things under the carpet. It'll go away if we leave it. Except they didn't leave it. When the family visit came, I was given a not very pleasant face-to-face ultimatum to leave the marital home because I was 'dead to them'.

I couldn't speak. I was not a confrontational person, so the wimp that I used to be left within the twenty minutes I had been given to gather my stuff together and leave! I don't drive, so after some hastily made calls to my company and one to my girlfriends, I left for an early start at work, but not until I had thrown the few essential possessions I had into a shopping trolley and a few carrier bags.

I had met my girlfriends, Alice and Mary, on social media months earlier. They were both transitioning. Mary, I had come to know from my work as a security officer. She used to deliver food goods to one of the other haulage companies I worked for. Often sharing cigarettes, we would chat about our respective situations. We got along so well that I met Mary's partner, Alice, and after many phone conversations and getting to know her, they asked if I wanted to visit them.

On the day I had to leave my partner, I rang the ladies, explaining about the change of circumstances. My visit was to become a few weeks but, bless them, they didn't hesitate. I heard the quivering emotion in my own voice as I explained about my need to escape, to get away, and just feel safe. I felt such absolute relief when they agreed to pick me up from outside work the following morning.

The haulage firm was literally on the way from my old house (it had never been home) and my ex-partner's place of work. What would happen if she saw me and stopped? Would she cause a scene? My girlfriends would be coming from the other direction and I desperately prayed they got to me first. They did. And I'd never been so pleased to see anybody arrive on time. No time for niceties, I threw my worldly goods into the back of their car and got in.

'Thank you for this, girls. Pleased to meet you both in the flesh at last,' I said, holding out my hand. I felt pretty stupid introducing myself, but added, 'I'm Raychel, and you may have just saved my life!' I didn't know what else I could say.

Looking at each other, they didn't take my outstretched

hand, but instead we hugged each other on the side of the road. And it felt so right.

Their home was comfortable; English hospitality at its best with loads of tea, practical advice, and two very adventurous cats. I was very much into self-imposed 'lockdown', because I had no intention of ever going out again, especially not in male clothes.

The morning after the night before was the first time, after a shower, that I met myself as Raychel in a mirror. (Now it's a lifelong pre-occupation.) Of course, I had no feminine clothes at all, so first I borrowed make-up, a wig, and some clothes.

You need some kind of plan put together if you are going to transition. Proper clothes are essential. (Don't 'wing-it' like I had to!) Alice provided me with a few loose-fitting tops and dresses, which she said would just about fit me. It took a while to find a suitable combination, and I remember how frustrated I felt finding out that lady's blouses button up on the reverse side from men's shirts. It's something I still have trouble with. Each change of clothing bought a sense of peace and relief. To think that the act of putting on a woman's clothes could make me feel so happy. Yes! I knew this wasn't just an exercise in cross-dressing. It was so much more than that.

Making my first (indoor) complete appearance, Alice and Mary then helped me to apply make-up, warning me not to cry as it would ruin all their hard work. I almost did, but I was holding myself together. I wanted to wear my new face to bed, but it had to come off to save spoiling the pillows. (How naive was I back then?)

## *On the 2nd day…*

I'd been fed a hearty breakfast of bacon and eggs, plus copious amounts of tea. I'd showered and had my first 'proper' shave before becoming Raychel again. Goodness, this was a long process, not helped by comments like… 'Hurry up, the shops will be closing soon', and girlish giggling behind the bathroom door.

Not being the type to hang around, Alice 'suggested' that while the weather was warm it would be nice to venture out. I soon realised that her suggestions always became a reality. However, I had misgivings about going out in public quite so soon. I needn't have, though. Alice and Mary were well known in the town and very outgoing. I had only to follow their lead… self-consciously at first, but it got easier.

So, though it was for the briefest of times, their home became my haven and I was sad to leave. I really wanted to move into the area to be near them, but I didn't want to rely on them any longer than necessary. And with the local council involved, I could only stay for a three-week 'holiday' period. So, after getting a change of name, and the girls treating me to a new wig – among other things – I needed to move on. They know that I will forever be indebted to them, and I will love them dearly as both friends and sisters, who saved my sanity and possibly my life.

## *October 2017*

Surprisingly, it was not that long ago that I began to take back ownership of my life, and saw a GP asking for a referral to a GIC (Gender Identity Clinic). I dared to start kicking back against all I had known before. Almost three years! It seems like an eternity, yet I was almost sixty-three. All the misery I'd known and kept hidden behind a mask of compliance and servitude, from the bullies at school to military service (why would I even do that?), tormenting myself with a lifestyle I'd hated. Had I left it too late?

I sure used to think I had left it too long. Would I survive the surgeries? Did I have the time to have those important assessments? I worry with each day that passes that I don't have a new ache that needs to be investigated. Like many of us, I'd believed that I was living a 'normal' life, yet I had no friends to compare my life with. To me, everybody else was living a 'happy-normal' life anyway. Stupidly, I even let the incriminating evidence of mirrors add to the misery I'd felt for such a long time. Outwardly male, inwardly fighting to become myself.

I learned how to pre-judge people, because at the time it saved me from having to get too involved with them. Looking back, it was like wearing a suit of paper that I could have ripped off if I'd only known how. I've so missed out on making good friendships. Instead, my head hurt with the questions about my belonging. Who was I? Why was I damned to spend my life feeling like a leper? What were my parents protecting me from?

I didn't think I would remember much about my upbringing but, since starting this journey, I have surprised myself. In many ways, I felt secure as a child. As a family unit, we always had a roof over our heads, were fed and clothed, but something was missing. I felt emotionally numb. Almost as if I wasn't wanted,

'If you can't say anything sensible, don't say anything at all.' Did you ever hear that when you were growing up? It used to go hand-in-hand with 'Children should be seen and not heard.'

It all felt like a crushing life sentence to me. A life of desperate loneliness and self-imposed isolation. You see, I was brought up to respect adults as figures of authority, but more unbelievably looking back, that they were always right. That sentence became my touchstone. The underlying meaning was as sacred as a passage from the Bible.

'Don't speak until you're spoken to.' My hands felt tied at a very early age. My mind was certainly screwed up.

I needed answers to unasked questions.

Then, three years later my sister was born.

Could I have been jealous? You bet I could. Although I never knew what it meant. At one time I must have been feeling so despondent that I had to run away from home to get the attention I craved. And guess what? Nothing changed.

No-one wanted to befriend me because I never learnt to interact with them. I've grown up just wishing that I had friends, but I just didn't DO friends. I used to look at people greeting and hugging other people in the street, laughing and joking with friends and neighbours. My goodness, how I envied them. Was I some kind of hideous Frankenstein? It would have meant so much if someone had shouted 'Hi' to me across the street. I never once got that. Thank goodness Raychel does.

I have been asked how my children have 'coped' with my transition. They have long since passed into fully-fledged adulthood now, all grown up, and a constant source of pleasure and surprise to me. When I began my transition, I feared that they would not accept me or speak to me. After all, I had deserted them many years before, and really I had no right to expect anything less than to be totally outcast. I more than half expected it, to be honest.

I felt humbled that, after what I had put them and their mother through, they were tolerant of me. I am so blessed that our relationships have grown to that of a slowly growing acceptance that is now shared with a new generation of my family. I find it difficult to write about them. It's hard, because whatever I say here won't be enough to express the love I have for them. It cannot ever do them justice to say how proud of them I am, that they have not just learned to cope but learned to LIVE in this world, and they have done it despite me not being in their world.

They are a testament to the fact that their mum has been their anchor and rock. I am blessed and privileged to know you. C

## *My first day out alone… At the shops*

Be extra careful and vigilant, because some of you will be tempted by the urge to splash out on loads of women's clothing and accessories, especially make-up. (Quick solution: Go with a friend who adores shopping but has less money to spend than yourself.) Try not to get tempted. It seemed that any loose change I had in my purse I'd spend on that new eyeshadow I liked the look of, or a blouse that I'd be too embarrassed to try on (I didn't want others knowing I was unsure of my size). My real problem was that I wanted to talk as little as possible, because I was only too aware that my voice then, as now, was deeper than a ship's foghorn at sea.

## *Later the same day. Still alone. My reward…*

For not spending all my money at the shops, was sitting alone at a table in an English public house. I've been doing that for most of my life (being alone that is, not sitting in bars writing), so I'm more than just a little used to it. It's second nature. That makes me sound like an alcoholic, but I'm not. However, I really fancied a drink, and on this particular night there were a few customers who might be regulars on first-name terms with the bar staff, and the conversation seemed pleasantly subdued. It was a working day. Monday. Most guys around here are retired. Workers drink from home, as it's not as expensive, unless there is a 'footie match' on a giant TV screen in the pub, then it's like a tribal gathering.

There was no 'big game' tonight. I picked this pub due to its location, five minutes' walk away from home. It was a cool, clear night – a welcome respite after the stifling heat of this year's endless summer.

I was getting my bearings. Inside were two pool tables, a dartboard, a state-of-the-art, wall-mounted jukebox, seating booths, toilets.

Very important. There were three:

One for HE.

One for SHE.

And one for disabled.

Always a good thing to know. There never seems to be quite enough of them, eh?

Apart from a lack of bar snacks, everything else seemed to be in order, which reminded me that I kind of needed to (order, that is). I couldn't sit there looking like I was 'casing the joint' while I cased the joint. After all, I came out for a drink. So, I sauntered my best feminine saunter to the bar.

'Medium white wine... Umm, do you have a Pinot? Please,' I ask (in my baritone voice) the young lady behind the bar.

Several aged pairs of eyes looked fleetingly at her, then turned to me to play spot the difference in their minds. I watched the almost imperceptible frowns before they turned back to their drinks. *That situation went fairly smoothly*, I thought, *no overt hostility, at least.* Then...

'One medium Pinot. That will be £2.70, please, sir... Sorry, madam!' she corrected. We smiled. Knowingly. We chatted girly things, and I went home a happy lady on that first outing... on my own... in a new town.

I had been feeling very nervous for most of that day about venturing out as a lone woman, because the pub did have a negative reputation and I was half expecting a 'welcome committee' armed with baseball bats and broken bottles jumping me when I ventured in. I needn't have worried. Although in my mind I didn't quite fit in, neither did anyone take any real notice of me. Even though the footpaths would feel safer lit by Victorian gaslights, there is always a certain apprehension about walking alone in semi-darkness for the sake of saving public money, particularly for women. I'm very aware of my surroundings; I feel I shouldn't need to, but don't all women go through this?

Now that I have started my transition, it's easier to interact. I consider myself very lucky and blessed that I've been able to call on family members (some support me; sadly, some do not), and likewise friends that I didn't even have sixteen months ago. This will be my biggest ever life adventure. Like my two girlfriends, I can continue to transition while seeking my own 'normality' and confirmation that I am a woman.

Today, my once shaken confidence is something that I am constantly working towards improving. I will be free. Yes, it will be hard work, but so worth it. I feel validated. And I feel loved. That's all I've ever really wanted.

## *A message to my younger self ...*

If I could go back in time and speak to my younger self, this is what I'd say to her:

The journey is hard, but it is worth it, however long it takes for you to achieve it. For you to walk out of your own front door with your head held high and a swagger in your step, just being yourself. It's such a wonderful freeing feeling. I know in my heart that you can accomplish this. You are stronger than you believe.

There's no need for you to hide yourself in your room any more, under the pretence of shyness. You know, there is a huge world of endless possibilities just waiting for you. You deserve so much to be a part of it. Now is the time to learn how to be true and to love yourself. Let no-one say you cannot, because I am here to tell you: YOU BLOODY WELL CAN! Don't waste any more precious time.

Observe those around you who are walking their walk to a better, more fulfilling life. Go seek them out! Learn who they are, learn from them. Wisdom is giving you the go-ahead. Wisdom is amazing. You will need to summon the courage to initiate conversations. It took me a long time to do that, because I was so busy looking at their faces and trying to read their minds before I realised that (spoiler alert) nobody, except maybe a magician, can read minds – and I'm no magician. Be mindful; don't overthink any situations. Trust your own judgement then jump right in. (Like learning to swim, and I haven't drowned yet!) You will be astounded by people's honesty and willingness to help where they can.

A lot of people can talk a good talk! But that's it. They have no energy left to put anything into action. They will suck any natural empathy and love you have for humanity, and leave a dry husk. You know what? You are better and stronger than that. Cultivate new circles of loving friends. Know them. Trust and cherish them. Little things, like remembering birthdays, and children's names, and favourite colours. I used to think all this 'stuff' was unimportant, but it's a part of the very essence of womanhood, being able to express your emotions and needs.

I have no idea why our lives take the paths they take, but I am ready to enjoy the next part of my journey on older legs and with a much wiser head. Yes, it took me a while to understand that people are so wound up in their own lives to really give freely of that time to others. But I finally figured it out. I didn't know what I wanted, and it all comes down to self-belief, and learning to love myself.

I want to really, deep down, feel it in my soul when I

can truthfully say, I am a follower of God, who guides my thoughts and words. I am whole.

*I am The Girl Who Refused to Quit.*

## Dedication

To my daughter Angela for her unquestioning love and support and my son William who found it hard to begin with. In the wider net, My Sister Sheila & Mum Pam. Families are like streams, too many to name them all, but the source of all is my God.

## About the author

Raychel is a kind, good hearted listener. After surviving military life and a period of homelessness she has turned her life around to work as a volunteer for CRUK and likes to help out in church activities. She can be a bit scatty, wanting, in spare moments of relaxation to try her hand at cross-stitch she bought a kit...without a needle.

Raychel's first love has always been the written word, she has written across most genres and mainly for enjoyment. This is a first attempt at Memoir writing which she describes as being "Much harder to write about myself warts and all" She hopes to become a mentor to other Transgender ladies of mature years and their Allies, of who, "with the best will in the world" during the early days of Transition may need guidance too.

## Contact

https://www.facebook.com/rayCH.paterson
https://twitter.com/Newhack58
https://raychelgrace.wordpress.com/ Site under review by
   the author.

# Shine a Light
## Natalie Jane

Good Friday, 1999, I was at work in the newsroom in Northampton, in the days when I was a reporter for a local newspaper group and had to work on the majority of Bank Holidays. I was sitting at my computer, trying to get ahead for the following week's edition and keeping myself busy, but my thoughts were elsewhere and not really on looking through the pile of press releases I was meant to be sifting through.

My mind was occupied completely by worry and deep concern for my elder brother Tony, who was laid up in a hospital bed in Rugby. My amazing, talented, inspirational, and loving big brother. He had unexpectedly become bed-bound when he couldn't get up on his own the day before, and this sudden restricted mobility was now under investigation. How could such a fit, healthy, and athletic 36-year-old be almost paralysed and suddenly lack any physical body strength? I kept thinking what the diagnosis might be, but I reassured myself that due to his age and level of fitness he would be fine. Perhaps it could be a muscle weakness in his back, or a trapped nerve due to an old sporting injury from his school rugby playing days that he'd been having physiotherapy for over the previous few months

The morning into the middle of the afternoon dragged, but at 2pm we were told we could all go home and start our Easter break. Instead of going home, I headed to St Cross Hospital with my mum, dad, and fiancé. On our arrival at the ward, Tony was sitting up in bed with a smile on his face, but looking slightly pained in his expression. He seemed pleased to see us, but little did we know that his smile was masking that he knew why he was in such crippling pain. I remember him reaching out his hand to me and I held onto it tight as he started to tell us that an earlier body scan had revealed he had a mass, and it looked like a form of cancer.

I didn't hear much of what he went on to say. I was in total shock and disbelief and I really cannot remember how my mum and dad also took the devastating news. I could hear that he was still talking, but my head was trying to process everything, and I became quite distant and detached from the harsh reality of what I was being told. I heard the 'C' word and then everything fell silent to me. How could I process this news? I felt numb, shattered, and truly heartbroken.

I started to think about losing him, and though I wasn't losing him that day, I was thinking of a shorter future with him than I had hoped for. I stood still for ages, unaware of the time that had passed between finding out the news to actually moving away to cry out of sight of my strong, brave, and ever positive brother. I was broken, but I knew I wasn't the only one affected by the news. My mum and dad, my brother's girlfriend, and my fiancé, were just having to process what they were being told, too. The stark reality is that nothing can prepare you for being told that a relative or a friend has such a condition, and I especially was not ready to lose my rock, my soul mate, and my number one protector and confidant. I kept thinking there must be some hope for Tony, as a young, very active, and healthy young man.

Life after this day was a series of hospital stays and day visits, tests and procedures for Tony, who was later told that the initial skin cancer had spread to his bones. Every possible treatment and new clever medical technique was given a try. He also joked about being like a human pin cushion as he was subjected to blood test after blood test, which meant he quickly got over his initial fear of needles and giving blood. Throughout the entire process my brother took detailed notes – not including emotions or feelings – about when drugs were administered and what other treatments and procedures were being tried and tested. These precise notes and timings helped him keep track of everything that was going on with his body and health, and were probably more detailed and actuate than any medical notes. He became his own record-taker to relay every detail to all his worried and concerned visitors, who were ever-eager for an update/progress report and, of course, some good news.

My brother fought long and hard for a total of six years, and always showed remarkable strength and courage throughout. When he had good days or weeks, he would take advantage of them and do bits of housework, and made sure his decorating and gardening plans for the house were not neglected. He kept smiling throughout and made sure he made the most of every moment he spent with his love ones.

He didn't stop there, either. He wrote to his local MP to see if he could get a new cancer drug trialled in Warwickshire. The drug was not a cure, but something that might have extended his life and ease his suffering in the later stages of the condition. Unfortunately, the postcode lottery for drugs was not on my brother's side, and the MP wrote back to explain that although he understood my brother's position there was no way to get the drug for him or the rest of the county's cancer sufferers.

Over the next few years, I got married to my then husband Jon and gave birth to our first son, Josh, in 2003. My brother also met my second son in 2005. However, Tony didn't get to know my youngster for long before he sadly passed away. My second son was born on September 21st and Tony got to hold him once at about three weeks old, before he died the weekend after that first meeting.

I believe to this day that my brave and courageous brother hung on to meet Cameron, and then knew he could be at peace. At the time he died, I was up doing an early morning feed, and the news and timing of his passing hit me hard. His death had a huge impact on me and my future happiness, and I don't believe I have been quite the same since. I'd grown up with him being such a prominent and important individual in my life – one I had come to admire and look up to, really relied upon, someone who was always there for me and loved me unconditionally. Tony never had any children, but I knew from the love he had always shown to me, his little sister, that he would have made an incredible father.

The gaping gap his death created was massive. The loss was immense to me, but I was off on maternity leave with my son, and he and my little family in Kettering were what kept my focus. Though I was broken and didn't really allow myself to accept Tony was never coming back or would ever be part of our lives again, my daily life had to continue. Life, as it does, ticked on and the boys grew older, and I actually shelved my grief in the end by keeping busy. But I did hurt for a number of years after Tony's death, and I found it really hard to find me again and any kind of happiness. Due to the walls of unresolved grief and a loss of such a close family bond, my marriage to my first husband ended five years later, in July 2010.

During all five years of my mourning, I was also dealing with another loss of a different kind. My mum had MS for several years before Tony got sick, and her health had been deteriorating over the years. My relationship with both my parents had changed as my mum became less able and independent, and more reliant of my dad as her full-time carer. My husband and I had moved to Kettering in September 2000, but my relationship with my parents became quite distant due to my mum's health. I was feeling very isolated and alone, with mostly my husband's family helping us with the house and childcare needs. This also put strain on family life and took a toll on my emotional state. All the stability provided by my immediate family unit was crumbling away from me.

In August to early November 2010, I was single and searching for some form of happy existence again. This came via my best friend Julie introducing one of her male friends to me. I fell in love with him and he started to take care of me, and we began to build a life together. Early into our relationship, my family was struck by yet another loss – the shock and sudden passing of my beautiful Auntie Pauline, my mum's younger and healthier sister, who passed away on New Year's Day 2011. It was another devasting loss of such a beautiful and kind soul, who had been taken from us without any warning.

This loss also impacted my mum greatly; she had not only lost her son, but now her little sister, too. Then her own health took its toll on her, and in late 2014 into early 2015 we watched my courageous and positive mum's quality of life diminish before us. It started with her inability to eat or drink by herself, and she ended up being fed via a peg in her stomach. In March 2015, she contracted an infection which she was unable to fight off, and passed way in my dad's arms on the morning of 18th March, 2015.

Now, no-one can prepare for you losing a parent at any age, and I was 38 and felt completely lost again. I felt very vulnerable in the world and confused. I felt I had lost the real connection with my mum a long time before when her MS had taken away her ability to talk and interactive with us. But not to have a mum any more left me with a feeling of being exposed. I felt child-like again, crying out to see my mum, wanting her to comfort me and make everything alright, like only a mum can. But she was not there.

At the same time, my dad, who had been tending to her every need for many years, needed me to be strong and help him though this terribly sad period. I kept wishing for Tony to be back alive or Auntie Pauline to help us out, but there was just me and Dad now to get everything sorted and organised for the funeral. Time stopped still once more, and my role in the family changed and evolved again. My ex-husband helped with our boys and he looked after them for a week whilst I stayed with my dad and helped sort out the house and all the formalities. Then the following week, my dad lived in our home in Kettering as we waited for the funeral to take place.

I do not know to this day how I got through those initial weeks after my mum's passing, and I do wonder where my strength came from to carry on. The funeral fell in the Easter holiday and enabled me to have more time out from the normal routine of work. That helped with my grieving process, but the first month was an emotional blur.

My existence over the next few years went on at a steady pace as we all adjusted to life without mum, and the boys without their grandma. But with amazing support from family and friends, I kept travelling forward and making the most of my life, spending time with the special people in my life, including some of my oldest best friends. With their help, I found my smile, and even got married again.

At the end of March 2019, I went to Nottingham with two of my oldest girlfriends, Julie and Vicky, for a girlie weekend. We were staying over to see Bryan Adams in concert as part of his 'Shine A Light' tour. It was a lovely couple of days of fun, chatting, and laughs, and of course we agreed that we would not leave it so long to get together again. We continued chatting about our next get-together in our WhatsApp group, but the following month our conversations became more serious as Julie's health took a turn for the worse. When she collapsed, we thought at first that she had just been overdoing it at the gym and worn herself out, but then a growth was discovered in her stomach and we were told it was cancerous.

During the next few months, we tried to keep her upbeat, as she had a lot of things to process with her ever-changing medical condition. We had daily updates from her hospital bed via our WhatsApp group. There was an operation planned and cancelled, and treatment that never happened. Then within 48 hours of being moved to a hospice on Thursday, 20th June, 2019, our lovely, beautiful, and kind friend Julie peacefully passed away, just 39 years old.

My heart was torn apart, and a darkness closed in on me. This most recent loss hit me so hard, especially as she had passed away with very little warning and not after a long illness. How could this young and such beautiful soul be taken from us like this? I was left in such disbelief and indescribable depths of new sadness. It was like a huge tsunami, and I was drowning from yet another loss. It made me feel so fragile again and uncertain of life once more.

At times I was finding it hard to breathe and it took me a very long to find my smile and positivity. How was I going to recover from this? All my insecurities came to the surface, and to be fair and completely honest, it made me lose my self-worth and purpose. Those closest to me just didn't know how to support or reach me, particularly my second husband who was going through his own issues with work at the time.

I will admit that I lost half a year of my life in a very dark existence, and in two very different personas. There was the outwardly positive, capable, and highly functioning mum, friend, runner, and work colleague, but at home and in my married life, I was on a downward spiral into a very deep rabbit hole of despair. I lacked confidence, I was trying to work out what my life was all about, I had increased anxiety levels, and was constantly questioning why I'd had to go through yet another loss.

It took many more dark episodes in my life, including separating from my second husband, for me to start taking back control and to be able to start rebuilding my existence, finding me again, and learning from the lessons that come out of loss.

I started to realise that the way I had been existing was wrong and that I hadn't been true to myself. I was not being kind to myself and not healing from all my grief, and therefore I wasn't living my best life. When I realised this, I began to see things more clearly, and for the first time in a long spell, the dense fog that was stopping me really enjoying and loving life was starting to lift.

What I have learnt during my life is that losses of various kinds have been quite prominent over my lifetime, and have shaped and moulded me into the person I am today. I am not bitter or resentful, but still loving, hopeful, and living my life to the full. But I have been looking for people to almost pick me up from my grief, and not everyone around us can help with this process, whether that be through a lack of experience or understanding of the grieving journey.

I have had to learn to cope differently and to remember that you only get one life and it is for living without limits. Since my losses, I have just lived in a different form from previous years, and life is never quite the same. Any moving forward since they have left is positive, and is something that can be admired and can even give hope to others.

Create a legacy for them in their memory. Face fears or loss head-on, as nothing can be quite as bad as not ever having those ones in your lives anymore. But be grateful every day they were in your life and will always remain in yours hearts forever.

Whether you believe they are with you still in spirit, or looking down on you and sending you signs of their presence, our loved ones are still influencing us in our daily lives and actions. When I started running as a hobby and to keep fit, the first 5K I did was a Race For Life in Northampton in memory of Tony; my first Coventry Half Marathon I did was for the MS Society, for my mum; and I ran my first 10k at Stanwick Lakes on the anniversary of my Auntie Pauline's death. And most recently, I ran a virtual half marathon for my friend Julie around Kettering, and raised more than £250 for Cancer Research in her memory.

When I run, I feel that those I have lost are always with me, spurring me on to the finish line, as I remind myself my muscle pain is only temporary and that what they went through was a lot worse.

What I have also taken from the sadness is that you can be defined by your grief, but being defined in the right way makes you someone that those people you have lost would be proud of.

## *A message to my younger self...*

If I could go back in time and speak to my younger self, I would tell her not worry as much about her future. Everything will work out for the best in the end, even though there is a lot of heartache to contend with.

Your journey through life from childhood through to your early forties will definitely not always be a smooth one, and you will have to overcome a lot of potholes in the road; some are actually more like sink holes, to be fair! But you will prove time and time again that you will not be stopped, and nothing is impossible to overcome.

People will question your sanity and wonder how you can keep smiling with all the losses you have had to face, coming at you from all directions and in all kinds of forms. I cannot pretend you will not be hurt, and you will shed your fair share of tears over your lifetime – some justified, others not so much.

You will grieve, and you must give yourself plenty of time to do so. However, remember the lessons that these losses have taught you about the amazing, talented, strong, and loving person you are. And remind yourself how those that are no longer with us liked to tell you how proud they were of all you have achieved against all the odds.

You will experience moments of total despair and darkness, but you will pick yourself up and dust yourself down. Then head into the next chapter of your life with a huge smile on your face, and total joy and endless love in your heart for life and living it to the full.

I am determined to make a difference in the future, and at 43 years of age this is the start of my next exciting chapter and journey. So, love life and embrace it for all it is worth.

I am strong and beautiful, and the next chapter of my life is going to be so fulfilling and full of love.

*I am The Girl Who Refused to Quit.*

## Dedication

To the memories of my brother Tony, my dear mum, my auntie Pauline and my best friend Julie, I miss you all so much, but you are my inspiration for always carrying on despite all the upset I have faced. Love you always and forever.

## About the author

Natalie lives in Northamptonshire, which has been her home for the last twenty years of her life. She has been described as 'inspirational, caring, strong and determined individual with a heart of gold'

When she is not running races, leading her C25K running group or taking part in various Parkruns, she can be found exercising at home, reading, journaling and blog writing.

Mission: Natalie is currently sharing her positivity with others through her daily blog on Facebook: 'Reflecting and Refocusing' which she hopes to develop further in the future to help others deal with the grieving process. Her future aspirations include becoming a bereavement counsellor for Cruise, who helped her greatly to understand ways to cope with her losses.

## Contact

Facebook: Natalie Jane
Instagram: Chattynat1019

Daily Personal Blog 'Reflecting and Refocusing' on
    Facebook
Email: Nataliejsears@aol.com

# Feel and Be Free

## *Beth Haining*

To the outside world, I appeared to be a strong, popular, and confident professional woman. At 68 years old, I had overcome many difficulties in my life and I'd always come through smiling. Nothing kept me down for long; I was a survivor. I had attended counselling and personal development courses to address childhood issues.

I'm a qualified Probation Office/Social Worker and Life Coach. I was also one of the founding members and CEO of the charity Global Harmony. Many of the women I had supported with depression used volunteering with the charity as a stepping stone. Their involvement supported them in gaining confidence and self-worth as they prepared for attending further education or employment. Along with other volunteers, we organised fund-raising projects, raising money to support an orphanage in Ghana. I, and at times other volunteers, also visited Ghana to support work already being undertaken there.

I was sorted! Wasn't I?

The reality was that, on the inside, I was falling apart. I was facilitating groups for people with depression and anxiety, but before a group I would put my mask on to support group members. One night, driving home, I felt tears streaming down my face, but I wasn't feeling any emotions; I was numb. The next morning, I couldn't get out of bed. My whole body felt like it was screaming with pain, the tears started again, and then the first sob broke. I cried and cried; it felt like I would never be able to stop. I have osteoarthritis, so I am used to living with pain, but this was different. This pain consumed my whole body.

The tears kept coming and I struggled to get out of bed. I felt so tired and weak. I didn't want to go out, and only wanted to see the people I knew and trusted. I felt like I had lost my way, and myself. My life had always been an adventure. I was always busy socialising, fund-raising, or working and supporting other people, listening to their problems, and helping them to gain control of their lives. Why on earth couldn't I gain control of mine? I felt battered inside and out, overwhelmed with sadness, and my brain felt as if it was completely frozen. Would I ever feel normal again?

My friends told me that I needed to look after myself and to start putting myself first. I had always put others before myself, but it was time now to look after me. I had recently had several traumatic experiences, but all my life I had carried on dealing with whatever life threw at me. So, why was this time different?

I decided to start writing a journal, and as I wrote, the anger and blame flowed out of me. I did not read the content immediately; I just let go of trapped emotions. One day, as I was writing in my journal, I felt anger build up inside me and it seemed to consume me. I felt like I was stuck in a dark hole. I went to the doctor and was prescribed antidepressants, but they didn't make any difference, and the emotions and the tears continued to flow.

When I read my journal back, I realised that I hadn't allowed myself to feel any emotions for a very long time. I had always coped by keeping myself busy and by thinking, *I am okay, I can deal with this.* I realised then that the anger I felt was due to being scammed and disrespected, but I had to acknowledge that I was the one who had ignored red flags, and therefore I had allowed people to take advantage of me. I decided the only way to release myself from the past was to let go of the anger and blame and start exploring where my responsibility lay.

I had lived with my partner for seventeen years, and had thought we would be together forever. When our relationship broke down, my heart was broken. We had set up a Community Interest Company, running therapeutic drumming circles and creative workshops, but shortly after we separated, circumstances dictated that I couldn't continue with the company, so I returned to social work. Despite these huge losses, I didn't allow myself to feel any emotions from the breakdown of my relationship or the closing of the business. In my mind, it had happened, and I had to get on with it. I filled my life by staying with a friend and working until I was exhausted.

Soon after this, my sister was diagnosed with cancer and had to have chemotherapy and radiotherapy. She was in remission for a while, and then we were told the devastating news that the tumour had returned. How are you meant to deal with that level of pain? She clung to me tightly and we sobbed together, frightened of what was to come, and concerned about how our mom was going to cope with the news. When we told Mom, she fainted, and her body seemed to shrink overnight.

The time I spent with my sister whilst she was so ill was precious; we talked at length and became very close. My sister died in hospital after we had sat with her for hours; my mom had gone home – she was worn out and couldn't cope with seeing her daughter die. Other family members were with me, but as my sister's organs shut down, I had to make the difficult decision to stop the treatment. It was a hard decision to have to make, but she was in distress and the doctor said it would be kinder to 'let her go'. Her last words were that she wanted to come home with me, and this still gives me comfort.

Part of my mom died when my sister left us, and she never fully recovered from losing her. Six months after my sister passed away, I had a phone call to say that my stepfather had died of a heart attack. He was eighteen years younger than my mom; it was a massive shock for us all.

I rushed to my mom and she collapsed in my arms sobbing. As I held her frail, shaking body, I knew I could never leave her alone. So, I sold my house and went to live with her. From the sale of the house, I invested £40,000 to ensure I didn't have any financial concerns in my retirement.

I invested with a man I admired and trusted. He was a coach on a leadership course I had attended, and I had attended several workshops he facilitated which were linked to the investment company he had set up. He showed me his name on the Financial Conduct Authority website, I had read the book he had written, and I had watched videos of him on African CNBC TV, advising people on how to invest. I had no concerns, because he was also my friend.

Whilst living with my mom, I worked part-time. I had a pension from the Probation Service, and I continued to raise money for the charity and saw my friends. Living with me was a different story for my mom; her structured life was gone. My sixteen-year-old granddaughter moved in with us, and our busy, chaotic lifestyle made Mom shake her head in amazement. My very presence made the house feel untidy. We managed, though, and had lots of laughs and shared special times together. Mom would often tell me to 'put my gadget down' (my phone); she didn't understand that I did a lot of work for the charity on it.

I had many friends in Ghana and stayed in touch with them. One day, a musician I knew said he wanted to introduce me to a music producer who was interested in supporting the charity. He sent me a friend request, and we began chatting. We talked for hours, initially planning how we could work together, but before long, chat moved onto a personal level, He seemed so interested in me, as if he cared. I realise now he was grooming me and that I was vulnerable because I was looking after everyone else and not taking care of my own needs. He had worked with famous dance hall/reggae artists and we planned to put on a show together. We laughed a lot and our plans continued to grow. I had travelled to Ghana ten times since 2006 to support projects, and yearned to go again. I followed my heart and arranged for my friend to move into my mom's home for six weeks whilst I travelled there.

When I arrived in Ghana and met the man whom I had been speaking to for so many hours, we seemed to click immediately. We laughed, and it seemed that our dreams ran in parallel. We organised the show together, attended lots of meetings, and went on the radio to promote the charity. We also spent a lot of time with musicians, which was all very exciting. As our friendship developed further, he asked me to marry him several times, and I said no. He was a lot younger than me, and I really wanted us to get to know one another more.

Five days before I came home, we attended a party, at which he announced in front of everyone that he had arranged our marriage and we were getting married the day before I left. Was this for real? I felt like a rabbit in the headlights as everyone was happy and congratulating us. I didn't know what to do. How could I turn him down in front of all his friends? Against my better judgment, I went along with the plans, suppressed my concerns, and enjoyed the excitement and celebrations. It was not until I spoke to someone when the marriage was over that I realised I'd been manipulated.

On my return home, my friend told me she was very concerned about my mom. Her mental health had deteriorated rapidly while I had been away. A few weeks later, my mom took an overdose and my granddaughter found her lying on the bathroom floor during the night.

The ambulance ride seemed to take forever; I have never been so frightened in my life. Thankfully, Mom survived, and after a few days she came home. She didn't remember anything and could not understand why she had been in hospital. She was referred to the mental health team, and a psychiatric nurse visited her at home.

A few weeks later, I heard banging coming from her bedroom and went upstairs to find her smashing up her bedroom. She had pulled all the clothes out of the wardrobe, and some of them had been ripped up. She had torn up books and thrown all of her ornaments on the floor. She was sobbing, kneeling on the floor like a vulnerable child. I put her into bed and lay with her, hugging and stroking her hair until she calmed down. The tears silently ran down my face as my heart broke for her.

That night, I woke up to hear what can only be described as wailing. I ran to my mom and found her sitting on her bed pulling her own hair. The wailing noise she was making seemed to be coming from the depths of her soul. I sat with her whilst she continued to wail and cry throughout the night.

The next day, the psychiatrist visited and admitted her to hospital. They found fluid on her lungs and she was admitted onto a general ward. I stayed with her for hours, but unfortunately my beautiful mom had disappeared. Some days she did not even know me; she was writing notes saying she was in prison and they were strip-searching her.

For several nights, the hospital rang asking me to come to the ward as they could not contain her. She was trying to smash the windows with her walker, throwing water over nurses, and screaming. I had a meeting with the consultant and psychiatrist, who told me she had dementia and needed more support than I could offer her at home. I can't describe the unbearable feeling of having to let her be moved into a nursing home, but those feelings had to be suppressed as this was out of my control and I needed to support my mom.

On some days, she cried to come home, other days she didn't know where she was. I went to see her every day until she passed away in her sleep eighteen months later, aged 92. It was a happy release for Mom; she had wanted to go for a long time. I felt empty and lost, but again I suppressed my feelings, and kept busy arranging the funeral and dealing with other issues going on in my life. I now had two granddaughters living with me, and I was supporting them with their life journeys.

When my feet finally touched the ground, my investment was due to be paid out. I had previously received £10,000 back, so I completely trusted him. So, initially when I could not get in contact with him, I was not concerned. However, I then realised he had blocked me.

I found his wife's details and I messaged her, only to find he had taken everything she owned, including her children, and was now living in Spain. We have reported this, but no-one is interested. I was distraught that I had lost all my money. My dreams to travel in my retirement were shattered, but more than that, I was in shock and felt traumatised that this man I had trusted had turned out to be a liar and a thief. I continue, with his ex-wife's support, to find ways to expose him.

During this time, I was applying for my husband's spouse visa. I paid for the visa and was sending him money, which he called an 'investment into the music business', as I believed this would be repaid as it grew. During the visa application period, I was still having misgivings and actually said to myself out loud, 'Put a stop to this and save yourself a lot of heartache in the future.' But then I told myself not to be selfish. If the marriage did not work, we could be friends and carry on working together.

The application was successful, and he arrived in the

UK. Three days after his arrival, his mask slipped. He was extremely abusive – verbally, emotionally, and financially. I could not believe this was the same person I had talked to for hours and had felt such a strong connection with. I was desperate to get back to what I thought we had, but the more I tried to please him the more distant and abusive he became. I realise now that I was seeking his validation, but in reality that was not going to happen.

I don't like labelling people, but to try to explain my feelings I have used an anonymous quote:

*'Do you know why it hurts so much?*
*Because you're mourning a fantasy.*

*In the beginning the narcissist wanted to know everything about you, your hopes dreams, your innermost desires, secrets and fears. Everything you were looking for in a partner and from life. They seemed to be the person you have been waiting for! The one attuned to your heart's every need. In the beginning they treated you like a prize, the best thing that ever happened to them. It felt magical, a dream come true. But they studied you, exploiting your innermost self to find your weaknesses. Then the dream becomes a nightmare as the person you trusted turns everything you shared into weapons. The higher they made you feel, the deeper down they make you fall. It hurts because to you it was real. You glimpsed your idea of true happiness; if only they had stayed the person they pretended to be – you would have what you had hoped for. There is a reason it seemed too good to be true; the reason it hurts so much is because you are mourning something that never existed.'*

Unknown

Of course, there is a lot more to this story, but I will just say that eventually he said he wanted to go back to Ghana, and I gave him his airfare home. He didn't return home, but I cut all contact with him. When his visa was due to be renewed, he tried to contact me through friends and sent me flowers so that I would support his application. When none of this worked, he reported me to the police, claiming I had assaulted him! I had to go to the police station and be interviewed, but no further action was taken as there was no evidence and it was clear he had done this maliciously. He had seen on the Home Office website, *'If you have been subjected to domestic abuse you might be allowed to stay in the UK.'*

Just before I was interviewed by the police, I was driving to a hospital appointment when a man drove straight into me from a side road. My car was a write-off, I suffered concussion and whiplash, and mentally I felt very low. Until then, I had felt safe in my home and car, but now I didn't any more.

After the police interview, I read my journal again and it made me take a deep and honest look at myself. I had seen the red flags all along, and I had chosen to ignore them. I had totally disregarded my own intuition.

The hardest part of my recovery has been understanding how I allowed myself to be so used and abused? Was it arrogance that I didn't believe I could be taken in? I accepted that I had rescued him over and over again. The people in my life were shocked when I broke down. They said, 'Oh, you will be okay; you're the strongest person I know.' But the truth is no-one is strong all the time. We are all a mix of strengths and weaknesses. I kept going and going, thinking I was invincible. I had not allowed myself to feel or even think for some time; I was in overdrive, and I could not allow it to continue.

I see all these experiences as lessons, and I thank the Universe for them. My dad always told me, 'If there is an easy way or a hard way, you will find the hard way every time.' At last, I'm listening, Dad. From now on, I will continue to work on myself, I will validate myself, allow myself to feel emotions as they arise. explore co-dependency, set boundaries, and love and look after myself.

I have made a decision to take back control of my life, and writing this book is part of my recovery. Thank you for sharing the journey with me.

## *A message to my younger self...*

If I could go back in time and speak to my younger self, I would want her to know: You were planned and wanted, your parents loved you from the moment you were born. Your sister was quiet and tidy; she did not push boundaries and never caused your parents any stress. They thought you would be similar.

However, when you arrived you '*rocked their world*'.

Your life was an exciting adventure, you were inquisitive, a risk-taker, continually pushing boundaries. Your family didn't understand your free spirit; they were frustrated, you exhausted their patience. You were often told that you were naughty, a nuisance, and that you would push the patience of a saint.

Your mom's life experiences meant that for her to feel happy, everything had to be 'perfect' in her world. She would withdraw and cry if everything wasn't how she believed it should be; you thought this was your fault and responsibility.

Your dad's life experiences meant the only emotions he was able to show were frustration and anger. You craved his love and validation, and believed his lack of emotion was because he did not love you. In your desperation to feel loved and validated, you believed your own thoughts which were that you weren't who they wanted you to be and that they did not love you.

The sexual abuse you experienced by a close family member was not your fault. He controlled you, telling you that no-one would believe you. This was powerful, as you already believed you were not loved, so why would anyone believe you?

The belief that your parents did not love you impacted on you for many years and led to your craving to be accepted. You spent many years putting other people's needs before your own. Until you love yourself, you will never know inner peace. To love yourself, you must live in your truth. Always remember, the truth will set you free.

I wish I had known that I don't always have to be strong; it's okay to be vulnerable. Your vulnerability is the essence of your soul. Being able to survive everything I have been through has shown me that although I love to support other people, I must love and support myself first. I now feel confident to set boundaries and love, respect, and honour myself.

I am a survivor. I am strong, I am vulnerable, I am love, I am me.

*I am The Girl Who Refused to Quit.*

## Dedication

To my amazing friends who enrich my life every day, my mom, dad and sister who are gone but not forgotten. My children and partners, my grandchildren Libby, Macy, Eden and Seren. Who all inspire me to keep learning and growing.

## About the author

Beth lives in Worcestershire she has been described as being an earth angel with a heart full of love and fire in her soul.

Beth loves being a Life Coach. When she is not supporting other's, she is working on her own continual growth and development. She is presently writing her own life story sharing her life experiences and learning. She loves spending time with family and friends, she is known as the networking queen as she has a passion for meeting new people. Beth is about to start voluntary work with a group based in Birmingham who raise awareness of how living with HIV is no longer a life-threatening illness.

Beth's mission is to show people it's ok to be vulnerable whilst we experience life's ups and downs. She wants people to embrace the fact that we never stop learning and how important it is to be in touch with our emotions. We must feel to be free.

# Contact

Email bethhaining1@gmail.com
Facebook Beth Haining
Instagram Beth Haining

# Tinnitus and Social Isolation:
## A Healing Journey

### Isabel de la Cour

What would you do if every sound you heard, including your own voice, crippled you with unimaginable pain? If two people laughing felt like a knife stabbing you in the head, or running water made you flee in agony?

That was my experience in 2016, and it turned my ordered world upside down.

I woke up on 23rd January feeling fit, well, and healthy. I almost skipped down to the cashpoint. But by 10.30am, my left ear was feeling funny, like a train was going through my head. I tried the divers' technique of breathing while pinching my nose, to equalise my ears, but it didn't help.

By now, I could hardly stand up, and had to prop myself up against the kitchen counter. I had tunnel vision, the light was blinding, and all noise became distorted and amplified, like the loudest possible sound from a nightclub's PA system.

I took a cab to the GP out-of-hours service. There was a baby in the waiting room making normal gurgling sounds, but I felt like it was trying to murder me. A doctor walked in wearing leather shoes, and every step sounded like a bomb exploding.

'Argh, stop! Stop walking!' I screamed, crying hysterically. 'Please, no-one move. Your sounds are killing me.' I covered my ears with my arms, and slid off my chair onto the floor like a rag doll.

They sent me to A&E, where I was prescribed steroids and anti-viral medication. I was surprised not to be admitted overnight, but was discharged with an emergency appointment at the Ear, Nose and Throat hospital the following Tuesday.

I lived alone and spent two terrifying days plunging further into illness. I had a fever and there was a constant thunderous, crashing sound in my head. And then the vertigo started. It's a strange, scary sensation. One minute I was standing in the safety of my living room, and the next I was pinned up against the wall, breathless and panicked, as though I were balanced on the roof of a skyscraper with a sheer drop in front of me.

I lost my balance and had to shuffle around, holding onto strategically placed furniture so that my legs didn't give way. Eventually, I scrambled to the sofa where it still felt like I was falling to my death every time I lifted my head.

The diagnosis was Sudden Onset Hearing Loss. Doctors compare it to a stroke or a heart attack in your ear. They don't know what causes it, and there is no cure. I was told there'd be no physical improvement, that the tinnitus wouldn't reduce, but I would 'learn to live with it'. Were they kidding?

The first two months were a blur of illness and sleep. I was given medication for the vertigo, and slowly my balance returned. But there is no medication for tinnitus or sound distortion.

Before that weekend, I was a bright, bubbly woman, living a normal 30-something London life. I had a demanding job in a local government policy department, and a full social diary, constantly going to restaurants, bars, theatres, and galleries. That life abruptly ended, and I became a hermit.

But even a quiet life at home didn't provide respite. I'd run out of the kitchen screaming in pain whenever the kettle boiled or water ran from the tap. Their noise was grotesquely amplified and would trigger excruciating tinnitus. Going to the shops was an assault course of pain. Buses roared past, cars blared out music, and people chatted loudly on their phones. Each sound was a punch to the head, leaving me seeing stars and clinging to lampposts to stop me falling down.

This sensitivity to sound was caused by a debilitating condition called hyperacusis. It's believed to be a problem with the way the brain processes sound, rather than a mechanical issue with the ear. The idea is that the sudden nature of my hearing loss confused my brain, and it overcompensated by wildly amplifying all noise. As if this wasn't bad enough, sound is processed in the same part of the brain that creates fear and panic. When the brain loses the ability to process sound in this way, it interprets noise as acute danger. I was living in a state of constant terror.

Hyperacusis is treated with sound therapy to retrain the brain's sound processing ability. I was given a CD of everyday noises to play throughout the day, and advised to carry on my life as normally as possible. I took this literally, and in April I re-entered my life with gusto. I went to my favourite café and even had a pub lunch with my brother. I sat with gritted teeth as waiters clattered cutlery and baristas frothed milk for cappuccinos. The experiences exhausted me, and I slept, passed out with fear, for days afterwards.

I even returned to work. My first day back in the office was an unmitigated disaster. I was given the assistant chief exec's office to work in, but the rattling of the air vent made me cross-eyed and confused. Every time I braved the open-plan office, I was bombarded by phones ringing, printers whirring, and the hum of people talking. I couldn't even go to the loo as the din from the Dyson hand-dryers floored me.

I burst into tears at the end of the day.

'I can't do that again. It was too awful,' I said to my manager.

'Okay. How about you work from home instead?'

'That would be amazing, but I'll still come in for meetings,' I said, eager to please and unable to admit defeat. 'It should only be for a few months.'

Little did we know it would be for the rest of the year.

Working from home wasn't much easier, though. I'd fly through simple, administrative tasks but was flummoxed by anything which required a brain. Necessary phone conversations caused the tinnitus to spike to agonising levels. After each call, I'd flop off my chair onto the wooden floor and breathe deeply to calm my body down.

My social life was no better. I tied myself into knots with every social invite, unable to accept my new reality or let friends down.

'Getting out will do you good,' said my best friend on the phone, trying to convince me to come to her birthday drinks. 'The weather is going to be nice, so we'll be in the garden. Your hearing copes much better when you're outside.'

It was true, the tinnitus evaporated into the breeze. I'd started to meet friends in the park, but only on a one-to-one basis, so I didn't know if the hyperacusis would also reduce when outside.

'It's not good for you to be cooped up inside all day. You need human interaction. It will only be a few close friends who really care about you. You can always go home if it's too much.'

I could see her logic. I desperately wanted to be with my friends and enjoy group dynamics again. This would be a good way of testing the water in a supportive environment. However, the idea of going was petrifying. Every bone in my body told me to stay at home, but I worried that not going to my best friend's birthday would push the limits of her understanding.

After weeks of agonising, I decided to go. When I arrived, about ten friends were milling around the garden, their voices heightened after a glass of wine. A stereo played gentle background music. By any normal definition, it was a sedate soiree, but to me the patio doors opened on to an impenetrable wall of sound. I ran away and hid in the living room. People soon drifted in to see me and the quiet room became the noisy heart of the party. I got irritable with my poor friends who just wanted to see me, and implemented a strict one-in, one-out policy like an aggressive bouncer. I cried on the bus home; the party had reminded me of everything I'd lost. Would I never be able to be in a group again? Or have a laugh? What was the point of socialising when, despite my friends' best efforts, I still ended up in pain?

After that, I simply said no to all social invites, except one-to-ones in the local park. It was a relief.

I also turned to alternative medicine, as I felt the hospital had failed me. Thanks to homeopathy, there were significant improvements shortly after the party. The tinnitus slightly reduced, enabling me to step out of acute illness. However, rather than rejoicing, my conscious mind began processing my six-month ordeal. I became increasingly disturbed by the sound of the tinnitus, and dark thoughts dominated my head. Did I deserve this torture? Was it punishment for something I'd done?

The five years leading up to the illness had been hard. I'd had three family bereavements, my mum had undergone an emergency operation, my love life was a mess, and I was unhappy at work. Local Government had been decimated by austerity and there were stressful restructures and an ever-increasing workload with ever-decreasing staff. Twice I'd been close to taking voluntary redundancy, but had chickened out at the last minute.

I now put every decision I had made, and every personality trait – good and bad – under the microscope, as I tried to figure out what had caused this awful physical state from which the doctors said I'd never recover. The isolation, living in virtual silence and chronic insomnia, meant there was no escape from the self-recrimination. In my eyes, I was a failure and the tinnitus was my punishment.

By the autumn, friends and family had grown tired of my bizarre behaviour. The invisibility of my symptoms meant they couldn't understand the hell I was living in, and I was told to be less melodramatic and controlling. My social circle reduced to a few relatives and three or four very loyal friends.

'I'm going to refer you to the psychiatrist,' the hearing therapist said at my quarterly appointment.

'Things aren't that bad,' I said, but she saw straight through my denial.

'I'll do it as a precaution. There's a six-month wait and you may feel better by then.'

Constant, involuntary exposure to loud sounds is a recognised form of psychological warfare banned under the United National Convention Against Torture. Ten percent of women with severe tinnitus attempt suicide. Yet there was a six-month wait before I could see a shrink? I couldn't wait for that. I was going to have to rescue myself.

~~~

Within the bleakness, I was changing in curious ways. How do you occupy yourself when being near any sound cripples you in pain? Lurking in the vaults of my memory was a faint recollection of doing a cross-stitch pattern. I was astounded when the idea popped into my head, as I didn't sew and didn't think I had a creative bone in my body. It proved to be a godsend. Sitting quietly doing embroidery transported me to a meditative state where my body slowed down, my breathing deepened, and my anxiety reduced. As the year went on, doing this simple, repetitive stitch awoke a creativity in me that I hadn't known existed. I'd seen myself as a practical, organised person, and structured my life accordingly, but I'd always felt stifled and unfulfilled. Maybe I'd been frustrated because I wasn't recognising my creativity.

I also began questioning how I worked. At home, with no-one watching over me, I could step away from my computer whenever I got stuck on something. I'd spend 15-20 minutes washing-up or changing the bedding, and found these mind-numbing activities unblocked my brain and the solutions came much quicker than if I'd stayed staring at the screen. Over the years I must have wasted so much time and emotional energy sitting at my desk trying to come up with the answers, when all I needed was to do some housework. It was an empowering realisation. I saw the unnecessary pressures placed on me by my office-based job. Maybe I was not only creative but also in the wrong career.

I researched health, wellbeing, boredom, and creativity, and learnt how they are connected. Boredom and menial tasks, such as washing-up, make new neurological pathways in the brain which generate both artistic and cognitive creativity such as problem solving and coming up with new ideas. This new-found creativity was also helping me to heal.

The nervous system has two states. The sympathetic nervous system manages the body's stress response (fight or flight), and the parasympathetic nervous system controls the body's relaxation response (rest and digest). The body's natural healing system only functions fully when the nervous system is in the relaxation mode. The hyperacusis, tinnitus, and exposure to everyday sounds, were trapping my nervous system in the fight-or-flight state and preventing my immune system from working properly. In the meditative state induced by my embroidery, the parasympathetic state took over and my body's self-healing mechanism could start working.

I had thought my reclusive behaviour and sudden love of embroidery were desperate attempts to cope, but actually my body was telling me it was what it needed to heal. Luckily, I listened. Remembering the cross-stitch pattern from over 15 years ago and the intrinsic feeling that I had to retreat from the world rather than follow the hospital's advice to expose myself to sound, were my body's way of forcing me to move my nervous system into a place where it could self-repair.

Rather than see the psychiatrist, in mid-2017 I quit my job and went to Hawaii, Australia, and India. It was such a victory. I spent a year living in India – one of the noisiest places on earth – immersing myself in Ayurveda, India's ancient healing system, and exploring my creative side through embroidery and writing a blog about my healing journey. The fact that I managed to live there for so long is testament to the human body's amazing ability to heal and the approach that I've taken.

~~~

I am writing this in April 2020 during the coronavirus lockdown, when the world is struggling with social isolation.

'I'm climbing the walls!' said a friend during the first week. 'How are you coping?'

'I'm absolutely fine. I've been isolated for four years,' I laughed.

While travelling helped me heal, my health yo-yoed, and I struggled to break free from the shackles of isolation. I'm not sure if I'd grown so accustomed to being alone that I subconsciously sought it out, or if my body just needed more time to heal. Either way, I spent months in solitude, wrestling my demons and loneliness.

'Christ, now I get what you went through. Help me, give me some tips.'

'Well, there were two stages. First, I fought it, which is probably what you're doing now, but then I let all my old worries and expectations go. I accepted and relaxed into the isolation. I couldn't see it at the time, but that's when good things happen.

'Use video calls, so you don't get too lonely, but make sure you allow yourself to get bored. Boredom is actually great. I guarantee new interests will bubble to the surface and you'll discover fascinating things about yourself'.

Part of me was relieved when the lockdown happened. I'd recently moved back into my flat and was beginning to rebuild my life. The tinnitus is now a faint hum and the hyperacusis is virtually gone, but I still struggle with the frenetic pace of the modern world. My energy levels have never fully recovered, and I've seen the positives in a slower, calmer way of living. I don't want to return to being under constant pressure, commuting for hours, being a slave to messages and emails, and never being able to spend quality time with friends and family.

I hope the lockdown gives other people the chance to appreciate slowing down, to discover their creativity and enjoy new neurological pathways forming in their brains. I'm excited that conversations have already started about the possible impact home working will have on the work culture. I hope greater value will be placed on the quality of our outputs and outcomes, rather than the hours spent chained to our desks.

The lockdown is giving me even more time in quiet solitude where my nervous system can put the finishing touches on healing. Hopefully, when the lockdown is over, the world will have recalibrated and slowed down just a fraction to make it kinder on our bodies, improve our work-life balance, and make it easier for those with physical limitations to play an active role.

I'm looking forward to living in and finding my place in that post-lockdown world.

## *A message to my younger self…*

If I could go back in time and speak to my younger self, this is what I'd say…

I hate to tell you this, but you're going to get really sick and have a life-limiting condition. But there might be a way to prevent it.

Alternative medicine has never crossed your mind because you've never been ill. However, illness is brewing within you. Disease forms when you're not at ease, when you're frustrated by your life and annoyed at how things have panned out. You have been masking sadness for years. You'll go to therapy believing it will help you process everything that has happened in your life, but that won't be enough to stop you becoming unwell. Alternative medicine, especially homeopathy, will aid the therapeutic process. It will balance your emotions in a way therapy can't. It will help you manage the emotional shocks that are heading your way and limit their damage on your body.

You've never been completely happy or fulfilled in

your career. You've changed jobs, hoping things will be different, but you've never questioned whether you're actually working in the right field. You are much more creative than you think, and you need to be in a more dynamic, inspiring environment.

If these preventative measures don't work because the illness is predestined or caused by another factor, this is what you need to do to get better faster and with less suffering.

You need to see an orthodontist to realign your jaw. You'll have to wear a dental brace, but it will be worth it. You must also surround yourself with alternative healers and learn from them. The modalities that will be most beneficial are cranial osteopathy, homeopathy, and Ayurveda.

You need to adopt a healing mindset. You must believe, despite the doctors' prognosis, that you will get better. Never doubt it. The modern approach is to push through pain and discomfort, eg: 'You have to show your body who's boss. If you have a sprained ankle, walk on it. If you have sensitive hearing, stand in a noisy building.' But this creates a conflict in your body which is not conducive to healing. Disease means your body is already in conflict; don't create more.

You need to surrender to the illness, listen to your body, and accept where you're up to. If you feel too ill to leave the house, stay at home. If someone asks how you are feeling, don't suppress your emotions and put on a brave face; tell the truth. Acknowledging the physical symptoms is not the same as giving into them. It's a temporary measure to enable your body to heal. You can bring everything back into your life when you're strong and healthy enough to enjoy them, but for now you need to retreat from the world and, believe it or not, you need to do embroidery.

This illness will push you and your relationships to the limit, but you will get through it, and afterwards you'll be more content.

I am strong, resilient, and resourceful.

*I am The Girl Who Refused to Quit.*

## Dedication

To fellow sufferers of ear conditions. There is hope.

## About the author

Isabel lives in north London, where she grew up. She is so close to being back to her bright, bubbly self and is at a crossroads looking for a new career path. Before her illness she was president of a public speaking group and hopes to give speeches about health and well-being in the future.

She is currently writing a book about her healing journey.

## Contact

Blog: rapunzeltinnitus.com
Email: rapunzeltinnitus@gmail.com
Twitter: @rapunzeltin

# Embracing Me

## Carmen Modglin

Hidden deep,
Seeking escape with
No way out.
Words with no voice;
Soundless,
Powerless.
Potential meaning remaining
Voiceless,
Worthless.
Unspoken thoughts, dreams, visions, plans, stories,
Rendered meaningless,
Covered.

Heart racing, palms sweaty, all I could think about was getting to the stage. If I could push myself through the crowd and get to the stage, I'd be able to jump the barricade and get up there and grab the mic. The nausea almost doubled me over and my shaky legs threatened to give out. The idea of pushing through the suffocating sea of sweaty people made me want to vomit. I set my eyes on the stage, and with a focused intensity that I never experienced in myself before, I marched forward, scared and determined. The message couldn't wait for my comfort. This was life or death.

Approaching the stage, the urgency of my message overcame my meekness and I thrust myself over the barricade, jumped up the front of the stage, and grabbed the microphone. The band was on their break; the timing couldn't be more perfect. I scanned the crowd for someone to lock eyes with, knowing that the connection would help me breathe and speak clearly. No-one noticed I was up there. I couldn't see even one person looking toward me.

I started speaking into the microphone, but I couldn't hear my words over the noise. I spoke louder and realized that no noise was coming out of me. Desperation rose, as I needed to relay this message to these people NOW. I attempted to shout. Nothing. A feeling of overwhelming desperation started to set in as I frantically tried to get someone's attention. Flailing my arms now, shouting as loud as I could, doing everything I could think to do, but no-one could hear me, not even me.


The alarm clock blared, and I shot out of bed in a confused panic. It only took a moment to realize I was in my bedroom and not on a stage. I felt sweaty and cold standing there in the early morning darkness. My heart pounded hard in my chest. I breathed deep, trying to let go of the anxiety of that awful dream. I hated that it was back. That feeling of helplessness that it brought would linger for days. It did every time.

It was Christmas Eve afternoon and I was alone in bed.

The muffled sounds of Christmas music playing and the giggling and the carrying on of my family downstairs carried through my closed door. Every once in a while, one of the kids would crack open the door to ask another question: 'Mommy, can I wear my sparkle dress to church?'; 'Mom, where's the cinnamon?'; 'Mom, I really want to put those cute shoes on the baby, but she keeps kicking them off!'; 'Mom, where are my pants?'

For the third time, my sweet little blonde-haired girl quietly came in and whispered close in my ear, 'Mommy, when are you going to start getting ready for church?'

'I'm sick, baby, I'm going to stay in bed today,' I muttered weakly.

Tears of disappointment rolled down my little girl's face. She's my child who doesn't like to be away from Mama. My youngest by birth, who had to make a quick transition from baby of the family, youngest of four kids, to being the smack-dab-in-the-middle child when we adopted her three younger siblings in the year prior. She is a sensitive soul, full of creative energy and a little mischief, and she has an understandably strong need for Mommy's attention.

My frequent out-of-state travel schedule for work in the past year had made her even more clingy to me. I wanted to get out of bed for her. I knew that she was probably feeling overwhelmed with the bustling of the crowd that is our family, and she wanted the comfort of me being there when she needed me. I knew that she would especially need me at church, and I felt overwhelmed with guilt that I could not overcome how I was feeling in that moment and force myself out of bed.

I just couldn't. It was as if all of my body was being held down by some invisible weight. My arms felt heavy to move, my legs were like a ton of bricks. The heaviness in my chest made it hard to breathe deeply. I couldn't even crack a fake smile to try to make my little girl feel a little better. She left the room, defeated and sad. I felt defeated and sad along with her.

I was bedridden for days at a time over the next five months. The days that I was able to carry on with normal life were a constant struggle to make it through. This was a crash of momentous proportions. Aching body, extreme fatigue, and a deep dark depression set in and consumed my life. An avid reader, I couldn't focus my mind to even read a single page of a book. As a home-schooling mom, I struggled to do even the most basic of tasks for my children. As a business owner, I let go of so many responsibilities, severed relationships, and let down a lot of people.

Numbness of mind, body, and soul overtook my life. Not yet ready to admit to myself and to the world what was really going on, I focused on the physical condition of my body – the fatigue, the aching of my joints, the loss of strength. I couldn't even make it past noon each day without crashing and sleeping the rest of the afternoon. I let the world go by while I lay my couch.

The only strength I had was mustered for my quest to find out what was wrong with me. A medical check-up showed nothing out of the ordinary, but there was definitely something wrong. It's not that I was oblivious to the fact that I was struggling with major depression. It was so bad that I had pretty much disappeared out of life. Friends and work colleagues had become worried. Maybe it was just easier for me to explain that I was struggling with some unknown illness and trying to get it figured out rather than admit that I just felt done with life and didn't know how I could keep living.

I found a doctor who had expertise in natural healing, and spent a boatload of money over the course of the next few months on various healing modalities. Adrenal fatigue was the likely culprit of my poorly functioning physical state, and so we focused on healing my adrenals through nutrition, supplements, and various therapies. Acupuncture became something I looked forward to every week. Lying on a bed in a dim, quiet room with soothing music, this treatment became more of a pampering session for me, a solace from the busy life I struggled to keep up with. The acupuncture physician became a sounding board as my pent-up thoughts would start to flow out during each session. One day, after assessing the effects the acupuncture had been having on my symptoms, this precious soul looked me in the eyes and said, 'Carmen, I know what we have been doing here has helped you in some ways, but I honestly think that what you truly need is healing at the soul level. I want to recommend a therapist for you.'

Those were the words that changed my life forever. This sweet, young acupuncture physician had no idea how her simple suggestion would set my life on a course of healing I had been resisting for so long that I couldn't even grasp that I needed it any more. After all this time of desperately searching outside of myself to heal my physical body, what I really needed was healing from within.

The realization that the last five hellish months of my life had been one long, drawn-out wake-up call was the beginning of freedom for me. The very core of my being was trying to make itself known. I had stuffed her down and hidden her for so long – pretty much my whole life – that when she decided to awaken, it was like a prisoner trying to break free. The physical breakdown was a purposeful torment. I knew in my heart what needed to be done, I had known for a long time. But I had been fighting against it with every ounce of strength, because I knew that in order to break free of this perfectly built facade of a life that I had created, I was going to have to destroy it.

Through the next several months of therapy, I realized that this feeling of being voiceless and powerless was so engrained in the core of my being that I had come to accept that constant feeling of hopeless defeat as normal. It was in my late teen years that I started have the recurring dream of being mute. The settings and situations varied, but the feeling was always the same – disconcerting, stressful, nightmarish. I had no voice. In the recurring dream, I always felt an intense urgency to relay some important message. I would get around the people who needed to hear the message, and when I started to speak nothing was coming out. No sound. I was soundless, mute, and I felt invisible. People weren't seeing me. They couldn't see the look of urgency and desperation on my face, the need to express what I needed to express. I was unheard, invisible, insignificant.

This dream came to me during times in my life when I felt pushed down, disrespected, put down. Unfortunately, those times were often. It also came to me during times when I felt my light starting to shine through and I was making my own effort to stay hidden, covered. Because no matter what, I needed to hide my true self. My true self was a little wild, when I needed to be the 'good girl'. My true self was opinionated and passionate, when I needed to be quiet and agreeable. My true self wanted to explore, travel, have adventure, when I needed to be satisfied with where I was. My true self was creative and self-expressive, when I needed to stay unseen and unheard.

I didn't feel like I could express anything that was inside of me, because I was afraid of not being accepted. I was afraid of calling attention to myself for thinking differently or that by chance I might express an opinion that was different from someone else's, then I'd have to defend that opinion and be different. I wanted to blend in. That had become my goal in life: to just blend in. But it was that blending in that led to the feelings of insignificance, and my willingness to continue accepting a life in which I was made to feel less than worthy.

There was always that little inkling that there was so much more to me than I allowed myself to be. Through those months of therapy, I dug deep, trying to discover the real me. I didn't know her. Why was she so elusive to me? I've always been extremely private, ever since I can remember. But I didn't realize that I was so accustomed to hiding myself that I didn't even know who I was. Why have I spent my lifetime hiding? Spending my life pushing down my own needs/wants/desires had brought me to a place that I could no longer exist. I had spent my life making myself small in order to avoid the conflict that asserting myself might cause. Keeping the peace is always easier.

Those dreams of muteness were an ever-present red flag to me that I was putting on some heavy self-suppression by silencing myself and allowing myself to be silenced. It just got bigger and bigger throughout my life over time, until it got to a point of absolute misery. I had allowed my desire for the approval of someone outside of myself to override my entire sense of self. I had made decisions in my life solely for the sake of keeping the peace. I had decided that walking on eggshells was better than the price I had to pay for asserting myself in any way. And where it got me was feeling trapped in a life I could no longer bear. I didn't even know myself. I didn't know my own likes and dislikes; I didn't know what my own dreams for the future were. I had accepted a life in a toxic relationship, and just accepted that that is how my life would be. Until I could no longer accept that.

The more expressive I became in my professional life, the more repressed my personal voice became. Despite my shyness and quietness, I did find ways to express myself in my professional life. I had transformed from a very shy and timid girl to a person who educated and inspired others. I had found a passion in helping moms be the best they could be, and had spent years building a career path focused on helping moms create a healthier lifestyle for their families. Starting off small helped give me courage to take that next bigger step. I found empowerment through my experience of becoming a mother, and I became an educator, teaching new mothers-to-be to trust their bodies through the process of birth. I found employment where I could continue this calling to help women be empowered through their birth experiences, and continued my education so that I could help in more ways.

Becoming an educator in that small intimate setting

of just a few women and their partners at a time, opened the floodgates and let my voice finally be heard. Each passing year brought new opportunities and new courage to stretch myself. I grew to love teaching and using my voice to teach and empower moms to bring health and wellness to their families. No longer did I feel scared to assert myself and express my ideas and knowledge. I craved more opportunities to do so and followed that passion.

However, the more courageous I became in speaking in my professional life, the more silenced I became in my personal life. It was like I had to shrink part of me to the smallest of small in order to allow the other part to grow. My world was confused. I was growing in courage and personal power, I was speaking and making my voice heard, I was a leader and an inspirer. I got to experience speaking to larger and larger crowds. Mostly small groups of a dozen or less, then 50, then 250, then 500, then 1500! But at the same time, I felt small and powerless and voiceless. Despite mothering seven young children, home-schooling, teaching, and growing a successful business, I was constantly reminded of all my failures, which reinforced the feelings of worthlessness and insignificance.

That Christmas Eve crash began my five-month final battle against myself to acknowledge the truth of my life. I already knew deep within my soul. I had known for a long time, but could not face what that would actually mean for my family. When I finally owned my truth, I had to accept that my life as I knew it was over. The embracing of ME, the honoring of who I am, the acknowledgment that I deserve better, and the refusal to continue to shrink myself for anyone else's comfort, meant that I would have to uproot my life and my children's lives and move forward as a single mama of seven kids. Owning the power within me made it impossible to stay where I was.

This is not a path I ever could have imagined for my life. I never believed in divorce. I've always been told that God hates divorce. I hate divorce. But here I am now, divorced. Children have a sense of knowing beyond what we often give them credit for, and one of my kids had asked many times over the years if I was going to divorce her dad. My answer was always a strong and confident, 'No.' That is, until it was a 'Yes'. What happened? Brokenness beyond repair. I always saw hope, always believed in change, always knew that healing could happen. But there comes a time when you have to realize that what has been, and what is now, very well probably always will be. And what if that is something that you can no longer bear? The thing about emotional healing is that not everyone will come along your journey with you. Some relationships need to be let go in order to move forward.

The work of therapy brought me to a place of self-acceptance, self-confidence, and most importantly self-knowledge. The most impactful words I have learned to say to myself are, 'I know my truth.' It took a while to find me and now I am committed to never losing myself again. Those dreams of being mute went away when I finally acknowledged and accepted myself as I am.

I let go of that striving to be who I thought I needed to be in order to be acceptable: the good girl; the perfect wife; the humble homemaker; the one who never rocks the boat. I have embraced the perfectly imperfect woman that I am. I have learned to honor my natural talents and abilities and not to compare myself to anyone else. I am uniquely suited to make an impact on the world in my own way. I learned that it is okay to want more in life. I learned that it is not wrong to want to shift from where you are to where you want to be. That you can always choose to grow and change and reach for the next thing in life, while being sincerely grateful for what you currently have. You can be fully content where you are and still know that there is more out there and be looking forward to it. And that is okay.

Life is good now. I have found strength I didn't know existed within me. I have found my voice, and I am no longer afraid to let myself be heard. Self-acceptance is freedom.

Afraid but determined,
Heart pounding.
Inhale the courage,
Exhale the fear.

Soul lifting from the deep
Breaking out of that tightly locked box
Breaking past the tangled twistedness
Lifting into the clear open sky.
Now unobstructed,
Unafraid.

Release,
Jump,
Expand,
Flow.
Flow to sweet freedom!

But
Back and forth she goes
For a while
While she grows in strength
Until it starts to feel normal to be
Brave
Fierce
Unashamed.

Standing alone,
Standing strong.
Not waiting or hoping for any outside validation
Not needing anyone's approval.

I approve of me
Finally
This is the Free Me
This is Me

*A message to my younger self*...

If I could go back in time and speak to my younger self, I would want to tell her that I know you don't know it yet, but you are pretty darn strong. Don't shrink yourself to make others comfortable. Embrace your strength. Harness that little flame that burns inside you, and fan it until it grows into the blazing fire that is you. Know that you walk in total freedom to be wholly and completely YOU at all times. The choice is yours. Do not seek the approval of others. Let your-self shine, and the people whose souls align with yours will show up in your life in unexpected ways. Allow yourself to dream. Dream your biggest dreams and go after them fearlessly. Don't settle for just good enough. You can be grateful for everything you have in life and still be looking forward to more! Take that risk, find that next adventure, follow your heart's calling.

I would ask my younger self for forgiveness. Forgiveness for not seeing my innate good-ness and instead only seeing my deficiencies and feeling like I had to frantically work to be better and to do better. I created a false belief in myself that I was not enough and never would be enough. I strove for perfection in every way – never reaching it, of course, which always reinforced my idea that I would never be good enough.

I wish I had known that we can never find fulfilment in the approval of others. Dear younger version of me, please know that your words and ideas are important, and people need to hear them. Do not be ashamed of your strong beliefs and emotions. That deep passion within you bubbles up and pours out because you have a purpose in life greater than you know. Keep writing and fearlessly share with the world what comes out of the depths of your soul.

Going through the things I have gone through has shown me that I am enough. I am uniquely created for my purpose in life. Once we can own our perfectly imperfect uniqueness, we have our power. Honoring our individual strengths and talents gives us the ability to shine fully. Let go of what you perceive as your weaknesses; no-one is perfect. Shine in your brilliance!

I now feel strong as I shed that lifelong habit of hiding myself, and now walk through life allowing myself to be seen and heard and known. I no longer shrink myself in order to make anyone else feel more comfortable. Now that I know and love who I am, I will never go back to that.

I am the woman who decided to stop muting myself in order to be accepted. The woman who decided that having a voice and speaking her truth was more important than keeping the status quo.

*I am The Girl Who Refused to Quit.*

## Dedication

To my children, Annabelle, Wesley, Landon, Juliette, Isabella, Jonathan, and Sara-Grace, who have given me the strength to keep moving forward. May each of you always know that I love you unconditionally just as you are, and may you always have the courage to be you.

## About the Author

Carmen is a natural health enthusiast, a mama of 7 children, a certified health coach, and a Wellness Advocate with doTERRA. She lives in sunny Florida, USA.

Carmen finds great joy in helping other moms transform their lives from "just surviving" to THRIVING! She mentors women who are on a path of creating abundant health and wealth for themselves and their families, knowing that when mama is happy, healthy and living abundantly she has more energy, light, and joy to share with her children.

In addition to doing all the mommy things and running her business, Carmen makes beach time, sunshine, and long walks with an audiobook in her ears top priorities.

## Contact

Email: hello@carmenmodglin.com
Website: carmenmodglin.com
Instagram: @carmen.modglin

# The Grief That Doesn't Count
## Cassandra Farren

If you were to look up the definition of 'grief' in the dictionary, it would tell you that it is a response to loss, particularly to the loss of someone who has died.

My mum is 74 years old and has advanced dementia. She hasn't died, but I have been grieving for her for the last five years.

My mum has always been a woman who is young and heart. No matter what she was doing in her life, she always wanted to have fun. I remember as a child that we would go on holiday to the seaside, and me and my sister would be cautiously waiting at the water's edge when my mum would run straight past us, into the water, dunking her shoulders under. She would always be the first one on the bodyboard! As my mum got older and had grandchildren, she loved going to the soft play areas. She would be the first one to slide down the astroglide, the first one to dive into the ball pit, and the first one to be chasing my children through the tunnels.

My mum has always been a very caring lady. She told me about a time when she was walking back from the town centre and saw an older woman who didn't look very well. She walked her to the health centre, got her an appointment, called the woman's daughter, and booked her a taxi home. Mum would always say, 'If you can do something that will help just one person, then you should do it.'

That is the woman that I love, and that is the woman that I've lost.

My mum was a teacher, and when she retired she began to get a bit forgetful. She started to repeat herself a lot, but she would say to us that she had relaxed her brain now that she wasn't working.

We suspected that there was more to it than that. Eventually, we convinced her to visit the doctor, and that was when we received the diagnosis that she had dementia. We received a letter and a leaflet – that was it.

My mum phoned me that night, distraught. Crying her eyes out, she repeatedly asked what she had done wrong. I calmly said to her, 'Mum, it's okay. I'm a bit forgetful sometimes, but unfortunately as we get older either our body starts to wear away or our mind starts to wear away. You can still have fun and live your life. You'll be okay, we're all here for you.'

It wasn't until I searched on the internet for dementia support that I found a forum which asked me the following questions:

Did I want help with the early stages of dementia? The middle stages of dementia? Or the end-of-life stages of dementia.

I stared at my laptop in shock.

## *End-of-life stages of dementia!?*

So that was how I found out that this wasn't just my mum becoming a bit more forgetful. This is how I found out that my mum had a terminal condition, for which there was no treatment and there was no cure.

Over the next five years, both of our worlds went from calm to complete chaos.

Mum had been a strong, independent woman, who was always out with her friends; she'd often be walking, singing, or dancing. She loved spending weekends away with my dad, or months abroad visiting my sister and her family in New Zealand.

But she became withdrawn, scared, and anxious. She could no longer speak clearly or get her sentences out. She became paranoid and snappy. I forgot what it sounded like to hear her laugh. She would come to my house, and instead of greeting me with a friendly hug, I'd open the door to find her standing in tears, snarling and sulking, saying that she wanted to go home.

She wouldn't let my dad out of her sight, so he lost his independence, too. We arranged companionship carers to give my dad a break, but they had to be cancelled after just three months. Despite my mum not having capacity, she shouted and swore at them, saying that she did not need a babysitter!

Mum went missing and we had to call the police. The usually smartly dressed woman went downstairs to 'make a cup of tea' before letting herself out of the back gate, and was found at 7am in her pyjamas and a pair of socks.

I was thirty miles away, trying to bring up my two

children on my own, trying to run a business, trying to work two separate freelance jobs to make ends meet, trying to support my dad emotionally, trying to update my sister who was thousands of miles away... all whilst trying to come to terms with the fact that Mum didn't know who I was any more.

## March 2018

The day when everything got too much was when my mum called me and had a panic attack on the phone. Can you imagine someone you love having a panic attack on the other end of a phone? That on its own was horrific, but added to this, Mum couldn't speak properly, she couldn't breathe properly, and despite trying my best to calm her down, she could not comprehend a single word I was saying.

I'll be honest, there was part of me that wanted to hang up. How are you meant to cope in that situation? It wasn't like I could ask my mum to hold the line whilst I called the dementia helpline and ask for advice! Thankfully, after ten minutes, I managed to calm her down. But when I ended the call, I completely broke down. I sobbed my heart out, alone, in my kitchen. I was screaming, swearing, and shouting, pleading for help. If you had seen me in this state, you would have thought that my mum had died.

She hadn't died, but I *was* grieving.

I wasn't angry with Mum; I was angry that dementia was ripping our world to pieces. I didn't know for how much longer I could be strong. I was trying my hardest to be the glue that held everything together, but in that moment, I had nothing left to give.

I could have made an appointment at the doctor's, I could have asked to be signed off, but being self-employed, what was the point? I could have dried my eyes, crawled under my duvet with a big bottle of wine to numb the pain. But again, what was the point? My children were 15 and 9; despite me losing my mum, they still needed theirs.

What I actually did was dry my eyes, put on a pair of sunglasses to disguise my puffy panda eyes, and walked to school five minutes later to collect my son.

When we arrived home and my mum and dad arrived at my house, I had to pretend that nothing had happened whilst I took my mum in the garden for three hours whilst my dad slept the entire time on my sofa.

It was then that I knew I had to have the hardest conversation of my life with my dad and my sister. I told them that I didn't feel it was safe for Mum to live at home any more, and that we needed permanent help. We had done all that we could: we had padlocks on every gate, alarms on every door, we even a GPS tracker in Mum's handbag. But she'd get up, walk defiantly out of the house, and not take her bag with her!

We were petrified that she'd be hit by a car, cause an accident, or go missing again. I was in a permanent state of anxiety, and was constantly checking my phone. I didn't dare go any further than an hour away from home just in case Dad needed me. We couldn't go on like this.

The first time I called the care home, I felt like a complete failure of a daughter. I felt like I'd let Mum down; I was betraying her and her wishes.

She had begged me never to leave her in a care home, and told me that she would rather die than be left in an institution. She made me swear on her life that I would never do this, but tragically, the woman whose wishes we were trying to honour, was gone.

Thankfully, the woman who answered the phone wasn't just the Customer Relations Manager, she was also an angel in disguise. Laura said to me, 'Bring your mum in for an assessment, just for one hour, and we'll take it from there.' The last question she asked me was what my mum's favourite biscuits were.

As I walked into the care home with Mum that first time, I was petrified. What if she kicked off? What if she screamed? What if she shouted? What if she cried? What if she suspected where we were? What if she hated me? What if she never spoke to me again?

I took a deep breath and told the receptionist that we were there to have a cup of tea with my friend Laura. When Laura appeared, she greeted Mum by her name, said they were looking forward to welcoming us, and that they even had her favourite biscuits – custard creams!

By the end of our cup of tea and chat, Mum wasn't screaming or shouting. She was singing her favourite song, *Dancing Queen*, at the top of her voice. So, what did Laura and I do? We joined in, of course!

## April 2018

That hour led to my mum going to stay at the care home for one week. And that week led to what was the hardest day of my life – when I collected my mum from the house where she had lived for 30 years, for the very last time.

I had to watch her say goodbye to her husband, innocently assuming that we were going to meet my friend Laura for another cup of tea…

When I left my mum in the safe hands of the care home, I expected to feel full of sadness, but to my surprise the feeling that came over me was relief. Mum was safe, and that was all that mattered. But that didn't stop my continued grief…

One week later, I walked apprehensively back into the care home, not knowing what to expect. How would Mum react?

I saw her in the lounge before she saw me. She caught my eye, gave me a huge smile, stood up, and held her arms out towards me. I made my way across the room towards the big embrace that awaited as my mum joyfully began to speak. 'I knew it! I knew you would come. I've been telling everyone about you. Come over and sit down.'

Oh, my goodness, what a welcome! I hadn't been expecting this.

'I want to hear all of your news. Tell me, how are you? And how is your mum?' she asked me.

*How is my mum? Did you actually just ask me how my mum is? I'm your daughter!*

'Err, yeah. I'm okay.' *Please let that be a one-off; please do not ask me about my mum again!* I used to feel frustrated that my mum only knew who I was for the first ten minutes of seeing me, but now I was wishing we could go back in time. Had she now completely forgotten who I was?

I wanted to get up and walk out right then. What are you

meant to do when you want to relinquish all responsibility and run away? But the thoughts rushing around my head didn't stop my mum from carrying on with her questions.

'Where is your mum today? What's your mum doing?'

I wanted to shout, 'YOU ARE MY MUM!' I've never had any training of how to speak to someone with dementia, but I have learned through experience that you never correct them, you don't raise your voice, and you don't make them feel inferior.

I dug deep for some much-needed strength, and forced a calm answer to come out of my mouth. 'My mum's at home, she's in the garden.'

I must have sounded convincing, as my mum was beaming a huge smile at me whilst her friends were keen to know who her new companion was.

'You didn't tell us you had such a beautiful daughter,' one said. 'You look so alike; you can tell that you are both related.'

Cue my mum staring into space like someone had told her that an alien had just landed in the lounge.

This wasn't meant to happen. My mum had always known who I was for the first ten minutes. She would usually greet me with a hug and tell me how happy she was to see me. She would always ask how the boys were. She would tell me what an amazing mum I was, and that she was so proud of me. It was only after that ten minutes or so that she would start to repeat her favourite childhood stories, not speak a lot of sense, and then speak to me like I was someone else. Even though it was always hard, I had always been able to cope because she knew who I was for those first precious ten minutes.

Where had that time gone? Where had my mum gone?

## *April 2020*

Unfortunately, there is no happy ever after to this story. My mum continues to decline, and I continue to grieve…

There have been times over the years when a small piece of grief has broken my heart, like the first time my mum couldn't remember how to put her shoes on; this strong, independent woman, who didn't need help with anything, allowed me to put her shoes on for her. Then there was the time when she got her house keys out but couldn't remember how to unlock her own front door. And the time when she forgot how to make a cup of tea. That's what mums do, don't they? They welcome you into their house and then make you a cup of tea… Not any more.

There have been the times when a large piece of grief has broken my heart, like the first time my mum asked me if had children, the first time my mum didn't know it was my birthday, and the first time my mum asked me what my name was.

I consider myself to be quite emotionally resilient, but there is nothing that can prepare you for these overwhelming and harrowing moments.

Nobody sees these moments and not many people speak about them.

Over the last two years, all of our lives have had to change dramatically. But what this has taught me, and what dementia has taught me, is the importance of living in the present and to stop waiting for tomorrow. So, last year when my best friend asked if I'd like to be a part of her son's naming ceremony in Edinburgh, without hesitation I said yes. That is ironic, because before mum went into the care home, I would have immediately said no. At that time, I was in a constant state of anxiety. What if Mum wandered off? What if Dad needed me?

But now, I was looking forward to the four-hour train journey; it was the perfect opportunity to proofread my book, *I've Lost My Mum*, for the final time. After one hour of the journey, as we pulled out of the station I heard a loud commotion in the carriage behind me. A woman was crying inconsolably. She was trying to explain to the train manager that she had got on with her husband, but just as the doors began to close, he had stepped off the train… and he had dementia.

The train manager asked her to sit on the chair in front of mine, and before she'd even sat down, I got up out of my chair and sat down opposite her. I reached out, held her hand, and said, 'I couldn't help but overhear what had happened with your husband. I can understand how worried you must be. I understand because my mum has dementia, and there have been times when she has gone missing.'

There was nothing I could do but to sit and listen whilst passing her some tissues and some water. The train manager returned to tell us, thankfully, that her husband had been found and that the station staff would keep him safe until she could get the next train back. There was a moment of relief that washed over all of us, but as we caught each other's eyes again, I recognised the realisation of grief and sadness.

The realisation that this wasn't just about what had happened that day; it was the realisation of what was going to happen from that moment on, and how their lives were going to change.

At the next station, we said our goodbyes. And as I looked out of the window, I caught her eye as she waited on the platform. As my train pulled out of the station, she mouthed to me, 'Thank you'.

When the train manager returned, he also thanked me, and kindly upgraded my ticket to first class for the return journey. I also received an e-mail from his manager, once again thanking me for my help.

But actually, the person that they should all be thanking is my mum. It was my mum who taught me to help others. That is why I have shared our journey, in the hope that our story can make a difference.

I ask you to remember not only the incredible woman who is behind this chapter – my mum – but also her inspiring message:

If you can do something that will help just one person, then you should do it.

## *A message to my younger self...*

If I could go back in time and speak to my younger self, I would want to tell that her that she is strong enough to deal with any life challenge.

There will be times when you question everything and come close to breaking, but no matter how hard it gets, you will always find a way. Trust yourself, know that you are always doing your best, and that is enough. You are enough.

You may lose your way and feel like nothing is going to plan. This isn't because you have failed; it's because no-one has ever walked this path before. You are forging your own way.

Being able to survive everything I have been through has shown me that I am a determined woman who is on a mission to make a difference in the world.

I now feel loved and at peace. I trust in myself, and I feel proud that I have given my life meaning by authentically shining my light.

I am worthy of the beautiful journey that is unfolding before my eyes.

*I am The Girl Who Refused to Quit.*

## Dedication

To Kieron and Lennie, thank you for being my inspiration never to give up.

## About the Author

Cassandra, who lives in Northamptonshire, England, has been described as "a gentle soul powered by rocket fuel!"

She is the director of Welford Publishing, the author of six books and a very proud ghostwriter. When she's not mentoring authors or writing life-changing books, Cassandra can often be found relaxing by a beautiful lake or having a dance party in her kitchen!

She is a Reiki master who has committed to her own journey of personal and spiritual growth.

Cassandra's mission is to create a new generation of heart-led authors who collectively make a powerful difference in the world one book at a time.

## Contact

E-mail: hello@cassandrafarren.com
Website www.cassandrafarren.com
Facebook group / heartledauthors
Instagram: cassandra.farren

## Poem by Cassandra

Your questions have now been answered,
You know the steps to take.
Don't be afraid; be true to yourself;
Have faith, it's not too late.

It's time to replace your tears with smiles,
The best is yet to come.
You've got this chance to live your life,
Your happiness has now begun.

Follow your heart and follow your dreams,
Have courage to take the right path.
Believe in yourself, maintain your pride,
You've already come so far.

Hold your head high, live life on your terms.
You can do this, it's time to commit.
Know that you're worthy, take one step at a time.

From

*The Girls Who Refused to Quit*

# Acknowledgements

I would like to thank all of the authors from The Girls Who Refused to Quit. I am honoured that you have trusted me to become a part of your journey. Thank you for bravely sharing your stories which I know will empower and inspire so many others.

Thank you to Guille Alvarez for taking the incredible cover photograph.

Thank you to our editor Christine Mc Pherson.

Thank you to Jen Parker from Fuzzy Flamingo for typesetting our book and designing our beautiful cover.

*Cassandra's books* ...

# The Girl Who Refused to Quit

The Girl Who Refused to Quit tells the surprisingly uplifting journey of a young woman who has overcome more than her fair share of challenges.

When she hit rock bottom for the third time Cassandra was left questioning her worth and her purpose. She could have been forgiven for giving up on everything. Instead she chose to transform adversity into triumph and with not much more than sheer determination Cassandra has now set up her own business to empower other women.

She is the girl who refused to be defined by her circumstances. She is the girl who wants to inspire other women, to show them that no matter what challenges you face you can still hold your head high, believe in yourself and follow your dreams.

She is The Girl Who Refused to Quit.

# *Rule Your World*

Reduce Your Stress, Regain Your Control & Restore Your Calm

Have you ever questioned why your head is in such a mess – even when your life appears to look so good?

You know something needs to change, but don't know where to start?

When she became a single parent for the third time Cassandra feared her head may become a bigger mess than her life and inadvertently began to follow "The Rules".

Sharing her thought provoking and refreshing personal insights Cassandra's 7 rules will help to raise your self-awareness and empower a calmer, more fulfilling way of living.

Combining relatable real-life stories, and intriguing scientific studies with simple but powerful exercises,

you will gain your own "Toolbox for Life" as well as admiration for this determined and strong woman.

Cassandra is living proof that when you reduce your stress, regain your control & restore your calm, you too can Rule Your World.

# Share Your World

How to write a life-changing book in 60 days

How many times do you need to be told, "You should write a book" before you finally believe that you could become an author?

Your heart wants to share your story, but your head feels overwhelmed; Where do you find the courage to start, how do you make a plan to ensure you finish, and who would really want to read about your real-life journey?

Cassandra has written a positive and practical guide for aspiring authors, who want to make a difference to the lives of others by sharing their story.

In her natural, relaxed (and brutally honest!) style of writing, Cassandra shares her simple tools and tips whilst letting you into her own inspiring, yet unlikely, story of how she became the author of three books.

Cassandra's uplifting guidance will empower you to Share Your World and write a life-changing book, in only 60 days!

# I've Lost My Mum

I've Lost My Mum tells the true, soul-baring, account of a daughter who wants to make a difference to those whose lives have been devastated by dementia.

Cassandra's raw and deeply moving journey shares her own struggle for strength as well as invaluable insights into this invisible illness. This heartfelt and compelling story not only provides a deeper understanding of this cruel condition but gives hope that it's possible to find peace when someone you love is lost between worlds.

# Contact Cassandra

www.cassandrafarren.com
Facebook page/cassandrafarren1
Facebook group/ heartledauthors
Instagram cassandra.farren

The Girls Who Refused to Quit is a collaboration brought together by Cassandra Farren who is the director of Welford Publishing Limited.

To be considered to become an author in a future Welford Publishing collaboration, please e-mail:

hello@cassandrafarren.com

Lightning Source UK Ltd.
Milton Keynes UK
UKHW021111160820
368296UK00006B/284